GoodFood
Low-carb cooking

10 9 8 7 6 5 4 3 2 1

Published in 2013 by BBC Books, an imprint of Ebury Publishing
A Random House Group company

The Random House Group Limited
Reg. No. 954009

Addresses for companies within the Random House Group can be found at www.randomhouse.co.uk

A CIP catalogue record for this book is available from the British Library

The Random House Group Limited supports the Forest Stewardship Council® (FSC®), the leading international forest-certification organisation. Our books carrying the FSC label are printed on FSC®-certified paper. FSC is the only forest-certification scheme supported by the leading environmental organisations, including Greenpeace. Our paper procurement policy can be found at www.randomhouse.co.uk/environment

To buy books by your favourite authors and register for offers visit www.randomhouse.co.uk

Printed and bound by Firmengruppe APPL, aprinta druck, Wemding, Germany
Colour origination by Dot Gradations Ltd, UK

Commissioning Editor: Muna Reyal
Project Editors: Joe Cottingon and Sarah Watling
Designer: Kathryn Gammon
Production: Phil Spencer
Picture Researcher: Gabby Harrington

ISBN: 9781849906258

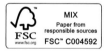

MIX
Paper from
responsible sources
FSC™ C004592

Picture credits

BBC *Good Food* magazine and BBC Books would like to thank the following people for providing photos. While every effort has been made to trace and acknowledge all photographers, we should like to apologise should there be any errors or omissions.

Peter Cassidy p35, p153, p167, p171, p177; Will Heap p59, p71; Lara Holmes p133; David Loftus p159, p191; Gareth Morgans p67, p81, p115, p137; David Munns p17, p21, p37, p41, p63, p69, p77, p101, p113, p125, p131, p145, p147, p151, p157, p175, p187, p195, p211; Myles New p19, p23, p31, p33, p39, p43, p45, p47, p49, p51, p55, p79, p89, p91, p93, p95, p97, p99, p103, p105, p109, p111, p117, p119, p123, p183, p185, p193, p199, p207; Stuart Ovenden p11, p15, p87, p189, p205; Lis Parsons p13, p29, p53, p57, p61, p73, p83, p107, p127, p141, p143, p165; Charlie Richards p173; Maja Smend p85, p149, p181, p209; Debi Treloar p161, p179; Philip Webb p25, p27, p65, p121, p129, p135, p139, p163, p169, p197, p201, p203; Kate Whitaker p155; Isobel Wield p75

All the recipes in this book were created by the editorial team at *Good Food* and by regular contributors to BBC Magazines.

everyday

GoodFood
Low-carb cooking

Editor **Sarah Cook**

BBC
BOOKS

Contents

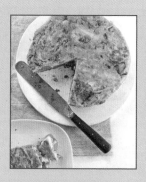

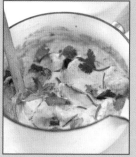

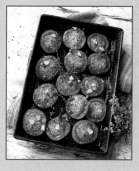

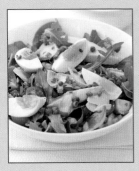

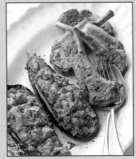

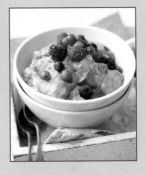

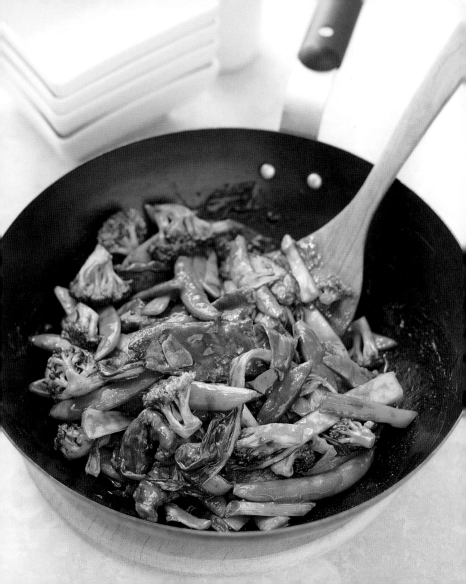

Introduction

Millions of people have had weight-loss success by following a low-carb eating plan but, let's face it, it can be as boring as any other diet, which is why we've created this fantastic little book for you. You'll find no funny ingredients or complicated recipes, just plenty of tasty, but naturally carbohydrate-light ideas, so you won't even notice that you're missing out. In fact, we've even added a few after-dinner treats just in case you're craving a mouthful of something sweet.

Each serving contains a maximum of 15 grams of carbohydrates, but most are much less – and many are low-fat or low-calorie too. You'll spot all the important numbers and nutritional analyses at the bottom of every recipe, so planning your meals is as easy as can be. And, as always, each recipe has been tested thoroughly in the *Good Food* kitchen – so you can be confident every one will be a success.

If you find your downfall is usually when there's something better on offer, worry no more. We've speedy breakfasts, simple weeknight suppers and a whole chapter packed with clever comfort-food classics you'd normally share with your family at the weekends – so you can still sit down and enjoy meals together. And if, like us, you're a real food lover and normally find diet food lacking in the wow-factor, we've also got plenty of options that are impressive enough for entertaining, so there's no need to cancel those dinner parties!

From sensational main-course salads that won't leave you reaching for the bread, to everybody's Friday-night favourite of fish and chips – this truly is a diet book with a difference. So, seriously, what are you waiting for? This book will bring back all the pleasure to cooking and make mealtimes something to look forward to again.

Sarah

Sarah Cook
Good Food magazine

Notes and conversion tables

NOTES ON THE RECIPES
• Eggs are large in the UK and Australia and extra large in America, unless stated otherwise.
• Wash fresh produce before preparation.
• Recipes contain nutritional analyses for 'sugar', which means the total sugar content including all natural sugars in the ingredients, unless otherwise stated.

OVEN TEMPERATURES

Gas	°C	°C Fan	°F	Oven temp.
¼	110	90	225	Very cool
½	120	100	250	Very cool
1	140	120	275	Cool or slow
2	150	130	300	Cool or slow
3	160	140	325	Warm
4	180	160	350	Moderate
5	190	170	375	Moderately hot
6	200	180	400	Fairly hot
7	220	200	425	Hot
8	230	210	450	Very hot
9	240	220	475	Very hot

APPROXIMATE WEIGHT CONVERSIONS
• All the recipes in this book list both imperial and metric measurements. Conversions are approximate and have been rounded up or down. Follow one set of measurements only; do not mix the two.
• Cup measurements, which are used by cooks in Australia and America, have not been listed here as they vary from ingredient to ingredient. Kitchen scales should be used to measure dry/solid ingredients.

Good Food is concerned about sustainable sourcing and animal welfare. Where possible humanely reared meats, sustainably caught fish (see fishonline. org for further information from the Marine Conservation Society) and free-range chickens and eggs are used when recipes are originally tested.

SPOON MEASURES

Spoon measurements are level unless otherwise specified.

- 1 teaspoon (tsp) = 5ml
- 1 tablespoon (tbsp) = 15ml
- 1 Australian tablespoon = 20ml (cooks in Australia should measure 3 teaspoons where 1 tablespoon is specified in a recipe)

APPROXIMATE LIQUID CONVERSIONS

metric	imperial	AUS	US
50ml	2fl oz	¼ cup	¼ cup
125ml	4fl oz	½ cup	½ cup
175ml	6fl oz	¾ cup	¾ cup
225ml	8fl oz	1 cup	1 cup
300ml	10fl oz/½ pint	½ pint	1¼ cups
450ml	16fl oz	2 cups	2 cups/1 pint
600ml	20fl oz/1 pint	1 pint	2½ cups
1 litre	35fl oz/1¾ pints	1¾ pints	1 quart

Blackberry compote

If you're picking your own blackberries, avoid any that grow on busy roadsides, and wash them briefly in cold water to remove any dust or bugs before eating.

TAKES 15 MINUTES ● SERVES 10
750g/1lb 10oz blackberries, halved
100g/4oz golden caster sugar
juice ½ lemon
small pinch ground cinnamon

1 To make the compote, whizz two-thirds of the blackberries with the sugar, lemon juice and cinnamon in a food processor until smooth, then sieve to remove the seeds. Fold the remaining fruit through the purée and eat within 2 days, or freeze in an airtight container.

PER SERVING 58 kcals, protein 1g, carbs 14g, fat none, sat fat none, fibre 2g, sugar 14g, salt none

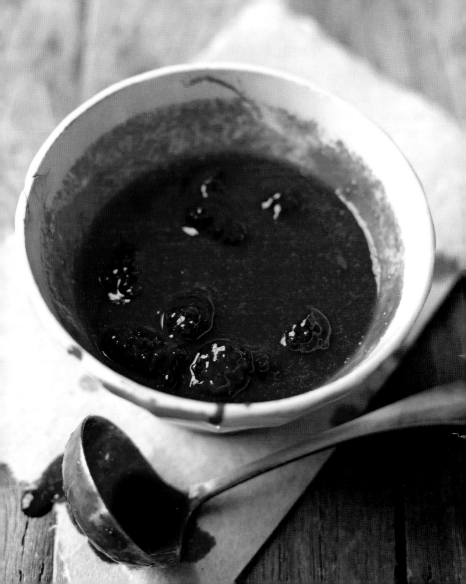

Cheese & ham souffléd omelette

This makes a great brunch or lunch, or serve it with a green salad for a speedy supper for one.

TAKES 20 MINUTES ● SERVES 1

50g/2oz Gruyère or Cheddar, grated
2 slices ham or gammon, roughly torn
2 eggs, separated
1 tsp Dijon mustard
1 tbsp chopped dill or basil
a little olive oil

1 Mix most of the cheese with the torn ham or gammon, the egg yolks, mustard, chopped herbs and some seasoning. Whisk the egg whites until stiff. Using a rubber spatula, gently fold the whites into the yolk mixture until evenly mixed.
2 Heat a splash of olive oil in a small non-stick frying pan. Pour the mixture into the pan and cook for 4 minutes until the underside is set and browned. Sprinkle over the remaining cheese and grill for 2 minutes until the cheese is bubbling and golden.

PER SERVING 507 kcals, protein 39g, carbs 1g, fat 39g, sat fat 16g, fibre none, sugar 1g, salt 3.48g

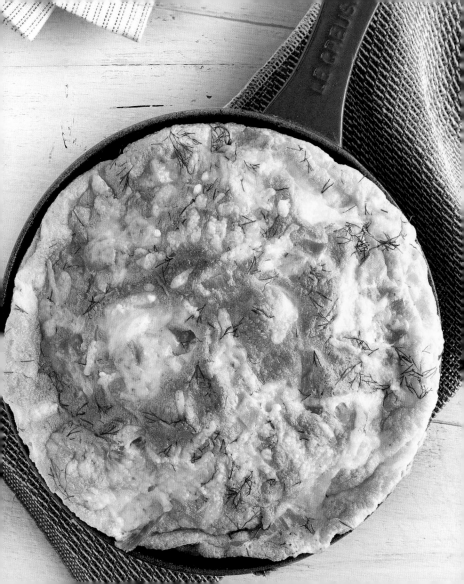

Veggie breakfast bakes

Packed with vegetables and very low in fat, this recipe makes it easy for you to hit your daily target of 5-a-day.

TAKES 45 MINUTES ● SERVES 4

4 large field mushrooms
8 tomatoes, halved
1 garlic clove, thinly sliced
2 tsp olive oil
200g bag spinach leaves
4 eggs

1 Heat oven to 200C/180C fan/gas 6. Put the mushrooms and tomatoes into four ovenproof dishes. Divide the garlic among the dishes, drizzle over the oil and some seasoning, then bake for 10 minutes.

2 Meanwhile, put the spinach into a large colander, then pour over a kettle of boiling water to wilt it. Squeeze out any excess water, then add the spinach to the dishes. Make a little gap between the vegetables and crack an egg into each dish. Return to the oven and cook for a further 8–10 minutes or until the egg is cooked to your liking.

PER SERVING 127 kcals, protein 9g, carbs 5g, fat 8g, sat fat 2g, fibre 3g, sugar 5g, salt 0.4g

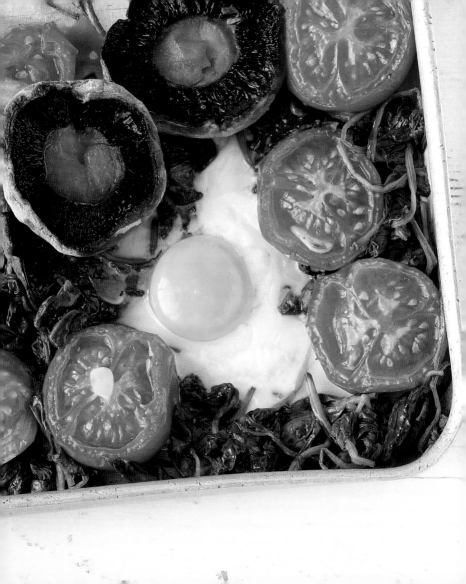

Energy bites

Grab one of these tasty treats whenever you need a quick energy boost, or serve as an after-dinner nibble with coffee.

TAKES 10 MINUTES, PLUS CHILLING
● **MAKES 8**

100g/4oz pecan nuts
85g/3oz raisins
2 tbsp peanut butter
1 tbsp ground flaxseeds (or try a milled
   seed and nut mix)
1 tbsp cocoa powder
1 tbsp agave syrup
50g/2oz desiccated coconut

1 Put the pecans in a food processor and whizz to crumbs. Add the raisins, peanut butter, ground flaxseeds, cocoa powder and agave syrup, then pulse to combine.

2 Shape the mixture into golf-ball-sized balls and roll in the desiccated coconut to coat. Put in the fridge to firm for 20 minutes, then eat whenever you need a quick energy boost.

PER BITE 204 kcals, protein 4g, carbs 10g, fat 17g, sat fat 5g, fibre 3g, sugar 10g, salt 0.1g

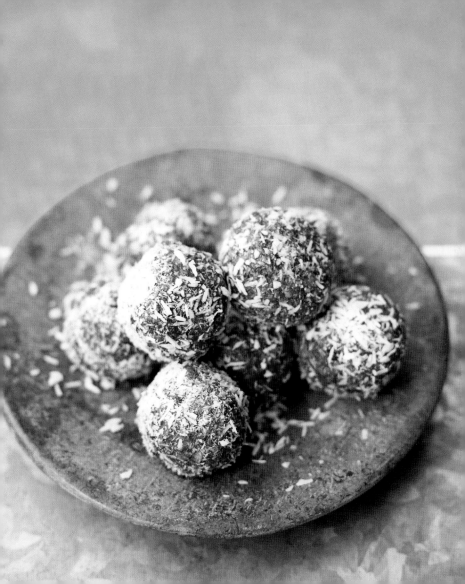

Smoked-salmon taramasalata

A great snack with celery and cucumber sticks. For a lighter version, you can swap the crème fraîche for low-fat Greek yogurt.

TAKES 10 MINUTES ● **SERVES 4**

100g/4oz smoked salmon
200g/7oz low-fat soft cheese
100g/4oz crème fraîche
juice 1 lemon
very large pinch cracked black pepper
drizzle olive oil
Kalamata olives and crudités, to serve

1 Tip the salmon, soft cheese, crème fraîche and lemon juice into a food processor. Blitz everything until smooth, then stir in the cracked black pepper.
2 Spoon the mix into a large bowl, drizzle with olive oil and serve with crudités and olives.

PER SERVING 203 kcals, protein 14g, carbs 2g, fat 15g, sat fat 10g, fibre none, sugar 2g, salt 1.8g

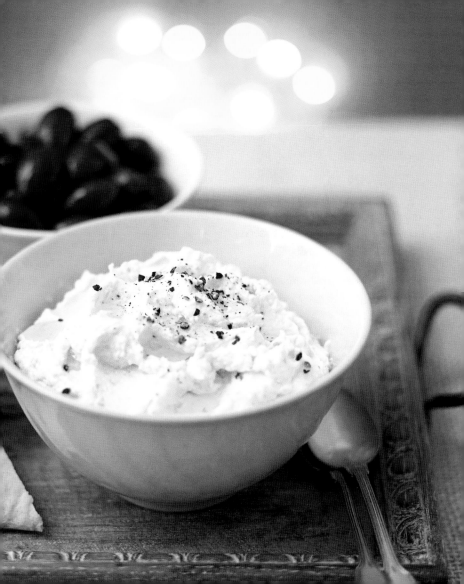

Green cucumber & mint gazpacho

This superhealthy chilled soup is perfect come summertime when cucumbers and avocados are at their best.

TAKES 20 MINUTES, PLUS CHILLING
- **SERVES 2**

1 cucumber, halved lengthways, deseeded and roughly chopped
1 yellow pepper, deseeded and roughly chopped
2 garlic cloves, crushed
1 small avocado, chopped
bunch spring onions, chopped
small bunch mint, chopped
150g pot fat-free natural yogurt
2 tbsp white wine vinegar, plus extra to taste
few shakes green Tabasco sauce
snipped chives, to garnish
few ice cubes, to serve (optional)

1 In a food processor or blender, blitz all the ingredients except the Tabasco, reserving half the mint and yogurt, until smooth. Add a little extra vinegar with the Tabasco and some seasoning to taste, then add a splash of water if you like a thinner soup.

2 Chill until very cold, then serve with a dollop of the reserved yogurt, a scattering of the rest of the mint and chives and a few ice cubes, if you like. The soup will keep in the fridge for 2 days – just give it a good stir before serving.

PER SERVING 186 kcals, protein 8g, carbs 15g, fat 11g, sat fat 2g, fibre 5g, sugar 14g, salt 0.28g

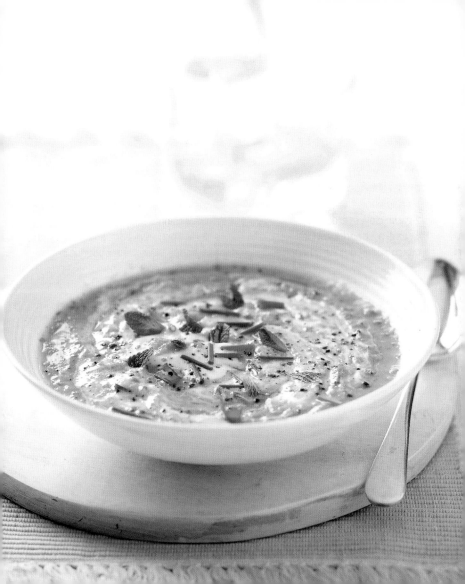

Prawn & fennel bisque

The prawn shells add a deep seafood flavour to this luxurious soup. Make and chill it a day ahead, or freeze it for up to a month.

TAKES 1½ HOURS • SERVES 8

450g/1lb raw tiger prawns in their shells
4 tbsp olive oil
1 large onion, chopped
1 large fennel bulb, chopped, fronds reserved to garnish
2 carrots, chopped
150ml/¼ pint dry white wine
1 tbsp brandy
400g can chopped tomatoes
1 litre/1¾ pints fish stock
2 generous pinches paprika
150ml pot double cream

TO GARNISH

8 tiger prawns, peeled but tail tips left on (optional)
knob butter (optional)

1 Shell the prawns, then fry the shells in the oil in a large pan for about 5 minutes. Add the onion, fennel and carrots, and cook for 10 minutes until the veg start to soften. Pour in the wine and brandy, bubble hard for 1 minute to drive off the alcohol, then add the tomatoes, stock and paprika. Cover and simmer for 30 minutes. Meanwhile, chop the prawns.

2 Blitz the soup as finely as you can with a stick blender or food processor, then press through a sieve into a bowl. Spend a bit of time really working the mixture through the sieve as this will give the soup its velvety texture.

3 Tip back into a clean pan, add the prawns and cook for 10 minutes, then blitz again until smooth.

4 To finish, gently reheat the soup in a pan with the cream. If garnishing, cook the 8 prawns in a little butter. Spoon the bisque into small bowls and top with the prawns, if using, and the fennel fronds.

PER SERVING 120 kcals, protein 7g, carbs 7g, fat 6g, sat fat 1g, fibre 3g, sugar 6g, salt 1.17g

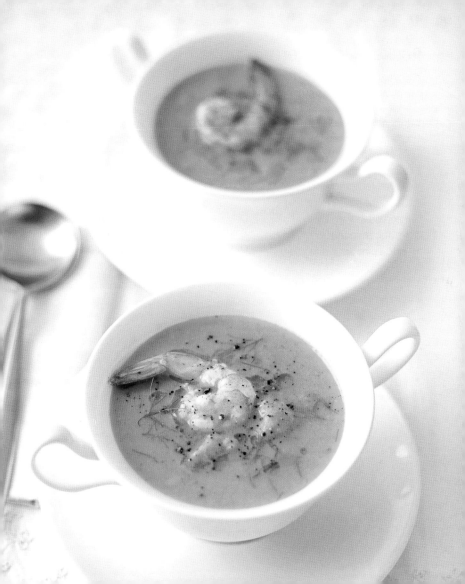

Rocket & courgette soup

This soup is a great way to use up a glut of courgettes if you're a keen gardener, and it freezes well, too; so why not knock up a double batch?

TAKES 40 MINUTES ● **SERVES 4**

1 onion, finely diced
1 tsp olive oil or knob butter
4 courgettes, grated or chopped
100g/4oz rocket leaves, roughly
   chopped
850ml/1½ pints vegetable stock

1 Cook the onion gently in the olive oil or butter for 5–10 minutes, until soft. Add the courgettes, rocket, stock and plenty of seasoning.
2 Bring to a simmer and cook for 5 minutes, until the courgettes feel soft. Whizz the soup in a blender, or use a stick blender, until smooth. Return to the pan and serve warm.

PER SERVING 62 kcals, protein 4g, carbs 7g, fat 2g, sat fat 0.2g, fibre 3g, sugar 6g, salt 0.7g

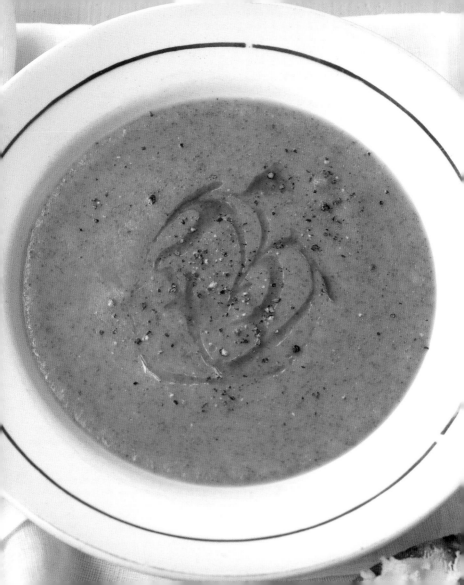

Asparagus with dipping sauces

Make one, or all, of these flavour-packed dips; when asparagus is no longer in season, roasted baby carrots make a nice change.

TAKES 50 MINUTES ● **SERVES 4**

24 asparagus spears, trimmed

FOR THE PARMESAN & LEMON BUTTER

juice 1 lemon

85g/3oz butter, cut into small chunks

25g/1oz Parmesan, finely grated

FOR THE ASIAN DRESSING

½ red chilli, sliced

1 tsp brown sugar

juice 1 lime

1 tbsp soy sauce

2 tbsp sesame oil

FOR THE GARLIC MAYONNAISE

2 garlic cloves, crushed

5 tbsp good-quality mayonnaise

1 tbsp olive oil

1 To make the Parmesan butter, tip the lemon juice into a small pan and, over a very low heat, add the butter. Melt and stir the butter into the lemon juice until you have a smooth sauce, add the Parmesan and season to taste, then set aside.

2 To make the Asian dressing, using a pestle and mortar, crush the chilli with the brown sugar, then stir in the lime juice until the sugar has dissolved. Stir through the soy sauce and sesame oil, then set aside.

3 For the garlic mayonnaise, mix all the ingredients together. Decant the sauces into three serving dishes.

4 Bring a large pan of water to the boil and cook the asparagus for 2–3 minutes until just tender. Drain well and serve steaming hot in a pile for everyone to help themselves and dip into the sauce of their choice.

PER SERVING (with all three dips) 431 kcals, protein 6g, carbs 5g, fat 43g, sat fat 16g, fibre 2g, sugar 4g, salt 1.42g

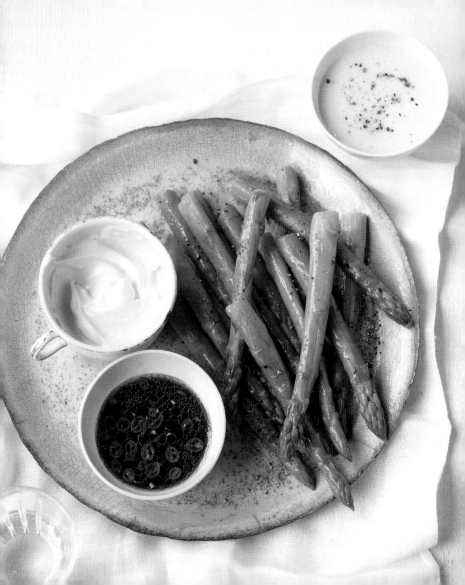

Amalfi-style prawns

This recipe is easily quartered if you're eating lunch alone – if you're throwing a party, double the quantities and serve these delicious prawns as nibbles.

TAKES 20 MINUTES, PLUS MARINATING • SERVES 4

2 tbsp extra virgin olive oil, plus extra for greasing
2 garlic cloves, finely crushed
12–16 mint leaves, shredded
450g/1lb raw peeled prawns
50g/2oz blanched almonds
lemon wedges, to squeeze over

1 Soak about 20 wooden skewers in water for 30 minutes. Put the oil, garlic, most of the mint (save some for serving) and prawns in a medium bowl, and season well. Toss to coat evenly, then chill and marinate for 1 hour.

2 Pulse the nuts in a food processor until finely chopped, but not ground – or chop with a knife.

3 Heat the grill to medium. Thread 3–5 prawns on to each skewer. Put the almonds on a plate. Shake any excess marinade off the prawns, then press the almonds all over.

4 Put all the skewers on a lightly oiled baking sheet, then put under the grill. Depending on the size of the prawns, cook on each side for about 2 minutes, until the almonds are golden and the prawns have turned pink. Watch them closely as they cook very quickly. Scatter with the reserved mint and serve with lemon wedges for squeezing over.

PER SERVING 217 kcals, protein 23g, carbs 2g, fat 13g, sat fat 2g, fibre 1g, sugar 1g, salt 0.6g

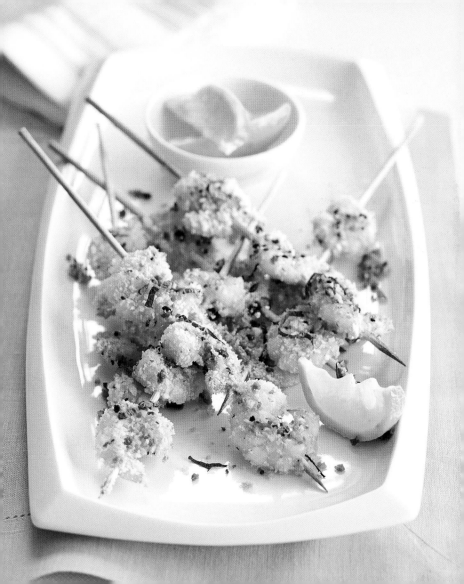

Turkey & ham salad

For a meat-free salad, replace the turkey and ham with 100g/4oz sliced chestnut mushrooms, 100g/4oz cooked green beans and 50g/2oz shaved Parmesan.

SERVES 4 • TAKES 15 MINUTES

180g bag mixed salad leaves
2 ripe pears
good handful walnut halves
3 slices each turkey and ham

FOR THE DRESSING

1 small red onion, finely chopped
1 tbsp red wine vinegar
2 tsp clear honey
150g pot low-fat yogurt

1 Tip the bag of salad on to a large platter. Quarter, core and slice the pears, and roughly chop the walnuts. Scatter the pears and walnuts over the salad leaves. Cut the turkey and ham slices into strips and scatter over the top.
2 Mix together all the dressing ingredients in a small bowl, then drizzle over the salad just before serving.

PER SERVING 240 kcals, protein 27g, carbs 14g, fat 9g, sat fat 2g, fibre 3g, sugar 14g, salt 1.67g

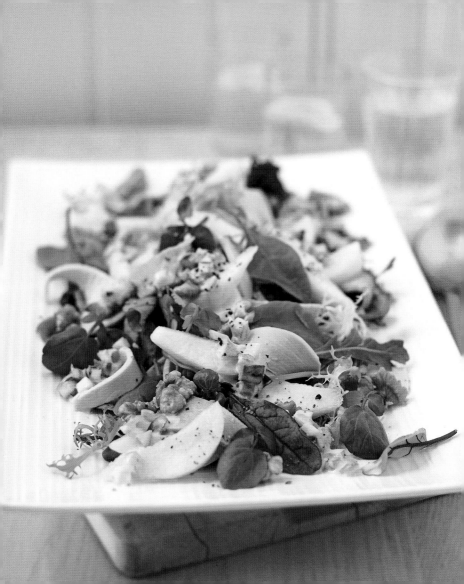

Prawn cocktail salad

To perk up ready-cooked prawns, refresh them in a bowl of iced water for 1 minute, then drain well.

TAKES 10 MINUTES FOR THE SALAD
• **SERVES 4**

200g/7oz large cooked peeled prawns
1 large ripe avocado, halved, peeled
   and sliced
200g/7oz cherry tomatoes, halved
4 spring onions, finely sliced
1 romaine lettuce, shredded
2 tbsp olive oil
juice ½ lemon

FOR THE DRESSING

3 tbsp mayonnaise
2 tbsp ketchup
juice ½ lemon

1 Whisk the ingredients for the dressing together in a small bowl. If the mix is a little thick, add a splash of water.

2 Put the prawns, avocado, tomatoes, spring onions and lettuce in a large salad bowl, drizzle with the olive oil and lemon juice and toss gently. Serve the salad with the dressing handed round separately.

PER SERVING 297 kcals, protein 14g, carbs 6g, fat 25g, sat fat 3g, fibre 3g, sugar 5g, salt 1.35g

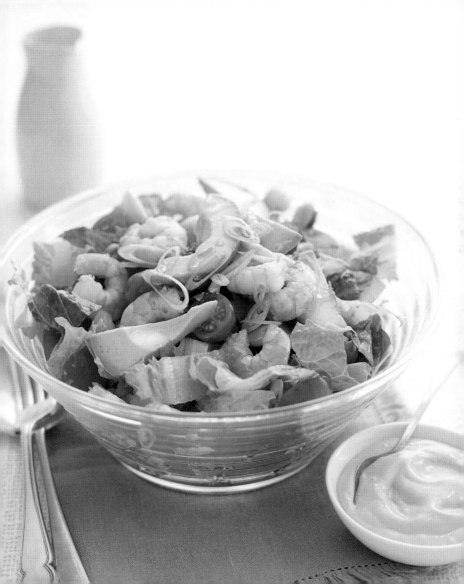

Pumpkin, halloumi & chilli omelette

A deliciously different way to liven up eggs. Cold leftovers, cut into wedges, make good lunchbox fillers the next day or a light lunch with a green salad.

TAKES 40 MINUTES • SERVES 4

2 tbsp olive or rapeseed oil
175g/6oz halloumi, sliced
500g/1lb 2oz pumpkin or butternut
    squash, peeled, deseeded and diced
2 red chillies, deseeded and finely
    chopped
1 garlic clove, finely chopped
2 tsp cider vinegar or balsamic vinegar
small bunch mint, roughly chopped
6 eggs, beaten

1 Heat half the oil in a large oven-proof frying pan. Cook the halloumi for 1–2 minutes on each side until golden, remove from the pan and set aside.

2 Add the remaining oil to the pan, then cook the squash for about 10 minutes, until soft and starting to colour. Add the chillies and garlic, and cook for a further 2 minutes. Pour over the vinegar, then put the halloumi back into the pan, scatter over the mint and pour on the eggs. Cook for 5 minutes until the base is set.

3 Heat the grill. Flash the omelette under the grill for 5 minutes until puffed up and golden. Serve immediately or allow to cool and serve cold.

PER SERVING 339 kcals, protein 21g, carbs 3g, fat 27g, sat fat 10g, fibre 1g, sugar 3g, salt 1.92g

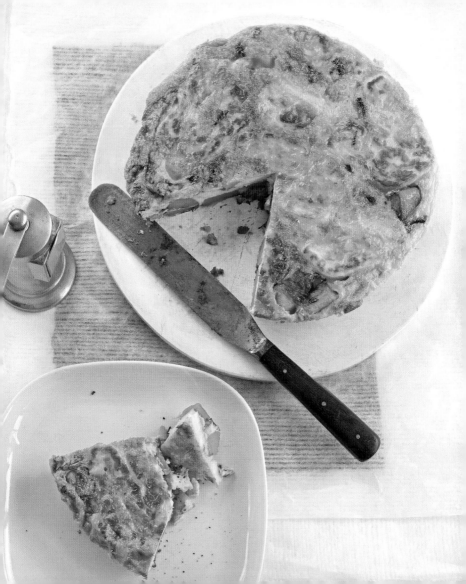

Goat's cheese, pea & bean frittata

Simple but satisfying, this is a great standby lunch that uses just five ingredients. If you don't like goat's cheese, feta will work just as nicely.

TAKES 25 MINUTES ● SERVES 4

300g/10oz mix frozen peas and beans
8 eggs
splash milk
100g log goat's cheese (the kind with rind)
1–2 tbsp chopped mint leaves

1 Heat the grill. Boil the peas and beans for 4 minutes until just tender, then drain well.

2 Beat the eggs with a splash of milk and some seasoning. Slice off four thin, round slices of goat's cheese (you'll use about half the log) and set these aside. Roughly chop or crumble the rest into pieces, then stir this into the eggs with the veg and mint.

3 Heat an ovenproof shallow pan, pour in the egg mix and gently cook for 8–10 minutes until there is just a little un-set mix on the surface. Top with the slices of goat's cheese, then grill until set, golden and the cheese is bubbling, and serve straight away.

PER SERVING 306 kcals, protein 25g, carbs 8g, fat 20g, sat fat 7g, fibre 4g, sugar 2g, salt 0.74g

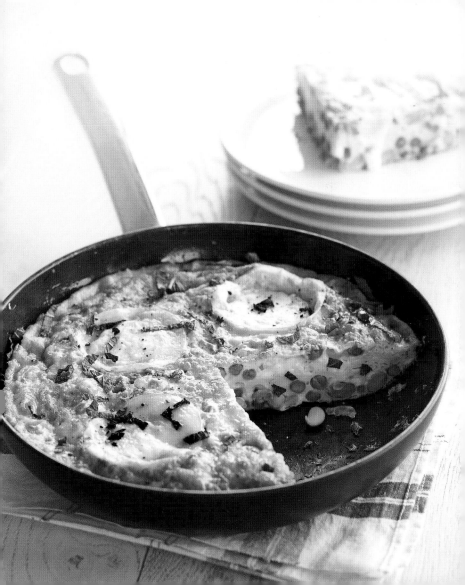

Fragrant Thai drumsticks

Delicious hot or cold. Marinate the chicken overnight before cooking, and the flavours will be even better.

TAKES 55 MINUTES • SERVES 4

2 tbsp sweet chilli sauce
grated zest 1 orange, plus 2 tbsp juice
1 garlic clove, crushed
1 tbsp good-quality Thai red curry
   paste
8 chicken drumsticks, skin removed
   and flesh slashed

1 Heat oven to 200C/180C fan/gas 6 and line a roasting tin with foil. Mix the chilli sauce with the orange zest and juice, garlic, curry paste and ¼ teaspoon salt. Add the chicken and coat really well.
2 Arrange the drumsticks on the foil, spaced apart. Coat the chicken with any marinade left in the bowl, then roast for 35–40 minutes until tender. Eat immediately or wrap in foil and pack up for a picnic or into a lunchbox.

PER SERVING 246 kcals, protein 31g, carbs 5g, fat 11g, sat fat 3g, fibre none, sugar 4g, salt 1.1g

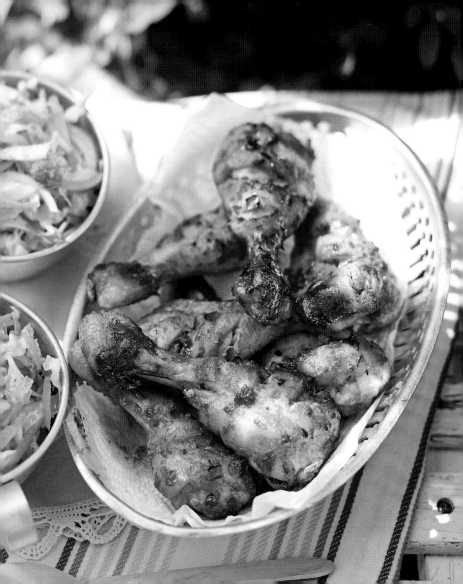

Turkish one-pan eggs & peppers

Vary this dish by flavouring the simple tomato sauce with whatever you have to hand – curry powder, pesto or fresh herbs.

TAKES 35 MINUTES • SERVES 4

2 tbsp olive oil
2 onions, sliced
1 red or green pepper, halved,
    deseeded and sliced
1–2 red chillies, deseeded and sliced
400g can chopped tomatoes
1–2 tsp caster sugar
4 eggs
6 tbsp thick creamy yogurt
2 garlic cloves, crushed
small bunch parsley, roughly chopped,
    to garnish

1 Heat the oil in a heavy-based frying pan with a lid. Stir in the onions, pepper and chillies, and cook until they begin to soften. Add the tomatoes and sugar, mixing well, then cook until the liquid has reduced, and season.

2 Using a wooden spoon, create four pockets in the tomato mixture and crack the eggs into them. Cover the pan and cook the eggs over a low heat until just set.

3 In a small bowl, beat the yogurt with the garlic and season. Sprinkle the dish with parsley and serve from the frying pan with a dollop of the garlic-flavoured yogurt.

PER SERVING 222 kcals, protein 12g, carbs 12g, fat 15g, sat fat 4g, fibre 3g, sugar 9g, salt 0.39g

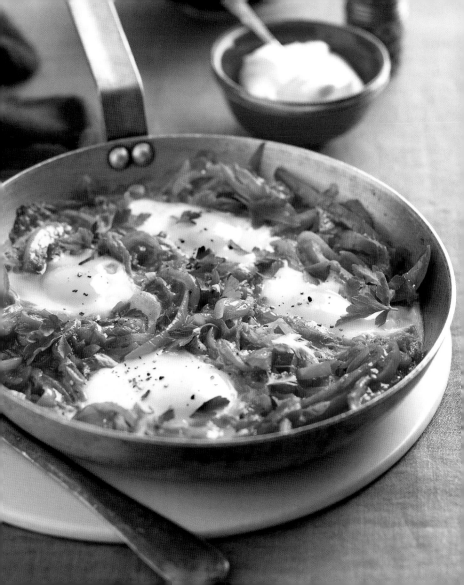

Halloumi with triple-crunch salad

For meat-lovers, why not replace the halloumi with chunks of chicken breasts marinated in a little harissa paste?

TAKES 20 MINUTES ● SERVES 4

2 tbsp white wine vinegar
1 tsp clear honey
1 tsp Dijon mustard
2 × 250g packs halloumi, sliced
1 tbsp mayonnaise
150g pack radishes, coarsely grated
150g pack sugar snap peas, sliced
lengthwise
½ cucumber, cut into thin batons

1 Make a dressing by mixing together the vinegar, honey and mustard with a little freshly ground black pepper – you don't need to add any salt as the cheese is quite salty.
2 Toss the halloumi slices in half the dressing, then griddle or barbecue for 5 minutes, turning until browned and crisp on the edges.
3 Stir the mayonnaise into the rest of the dressing, then toss through the radishes, peas and cucumber. Serve with the warm halloumi.

PER SERVING 438 kcals, protein 27g, carbs 5g, fat 34g, sat fat 19g, fibre 1g, sugar 5g, salt 4.73g

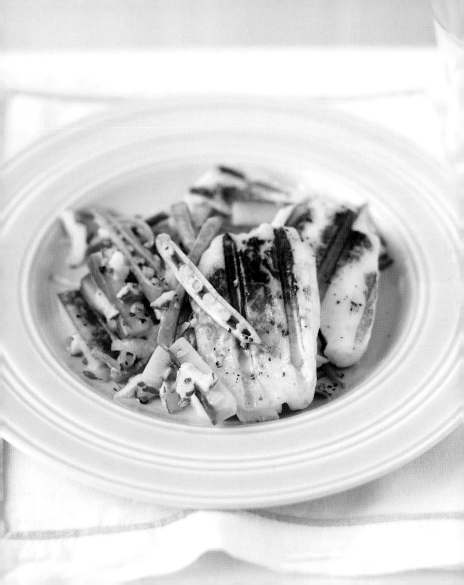

Sausages with oregano, mushrooms & olives

Sausages get the Italian treatment with this supertasty one-pan the whole family will love.

TAKES 30 MINUTES • SERVES 4

450g pack reduced-fat sausages
1 tsp sunflower oil
2 tsp dried oregano
2 garlic cloves, sliced
400g can cherry or chopped tomatoes
200ml/7fl oz beef stock
100g/4oz pitted black olives in brine
500g pack mushrooms, thickly sliced

1 Using kitchen scissors, snip the sausages into meatball-size pieces. Heat a large frying pan and fry the pieces in the oil for about 5 minutes until golden all over. Add the oregano and garlic, fry for 1 minute more, then tip in the tomatoes, stock, olives and mushrooms.
2 Simmer for 15 minutes until the sausages are cooked through and the sauce has reduced a little.

PER SERVING 264 kcals, protein 20g, carbs 12g, fat 16g, sat fat 4g, fibre 4g, sugar 4g, salt 2.19g

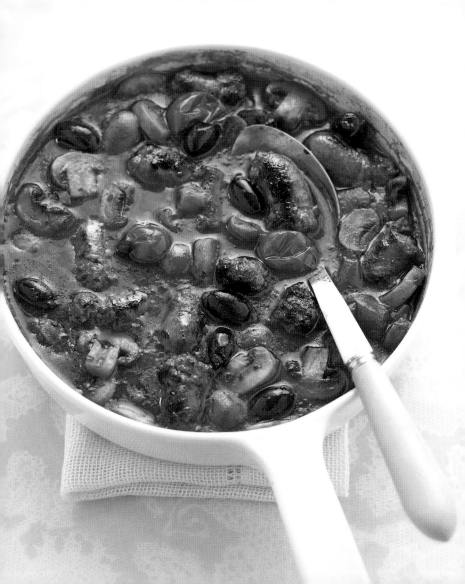

Trout with almonds & red pepper

Trout is quick and easy to cook, and makes a great heart-healthy meal.

TAKES ABOUT 40 MINUTES

● **SERVES 2**

1 large red pepper, deseeded and
    chopped
2 large tomatoes, roughly chopped, or
    handful cherry tomatoes, halved
1 garlic clove, chopped
1 tbsp olive oil, plus a little extra
1 tbsp balsamic vinegar
2 trout fillets (about 140g/5oz each)
2 tbsp flaked almonds
lemon wedges and rocket salad,
    to serve

1 Heat oven to 190C/170C fan/gas 5.
Tip the pepper, tomatoes, garlic, oil and
vinegar into a roasting tin, then toss
them together. Roast for 20 minutes,
then make a space in the roasting tin for
the trout fillets, scattering with the
almonds and a little salt and freshly
ground black pepper.

2 Return to the oven for a further
10–15 minutes, until the fish is cooked
and the almonds lightly toasted. Serve
with lemon wedges for squeezing over
and a rocket salad on the side.

PER SERVING 326 kcals, protein 31g, carbs 11g,
fat 18g, sat fat 3g, fibre 3g, sugar 11g, salt 0.24g

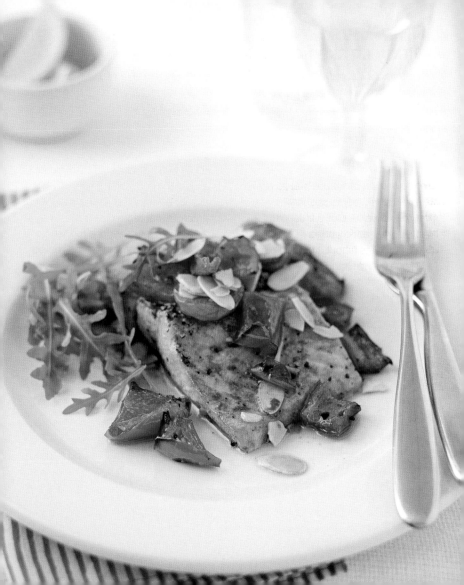

Nutty chicken curry

Fast and flavoursome, this creamy chicken curry is ready in under 20 minutes.

TAKES 18 MINUTES ● **SERVES 4**

1 large red chilli, deseeded

½ finger-length piece ginger, roughly
   chopped

1 fat garlic clove

small bunch coriander, stalks roughly
   chopped, leaves picked

1 tbsp sunflower oil

4 skinless chicken breasts, cut into
   chunks

5 tbsp peanut butter

150ml/¼ pint chicken stock

200g tub Greek yogurt

1 Finely slice a quarter of the chilli, then put the rest in a food processor with the ginger, garlic, coriander stalks and one-third of the leaves. Whizz to a rough paste with a splash of water, if needed.

2 Heat the oil in a frying pan, then quickly brown the chicken chunks for 1 minute. Stir in the chilli paste for another minute, then add the peanut butter, stock and yogurt. When the sauce is gently bubbling, cook for 10 minutes until the chicken is just cooked through and the sauce has thickened.

3 Stir in most of the remaining coriander leaves, then scatter the rest on top with the reserved chilli. Eat with mashed sweet potato.

PER SERVING 358 kcals, protein 43g, carbs 4g, fat 19g, sat fat 6g, fibre 1g, sugar 3g, salt 0.66g

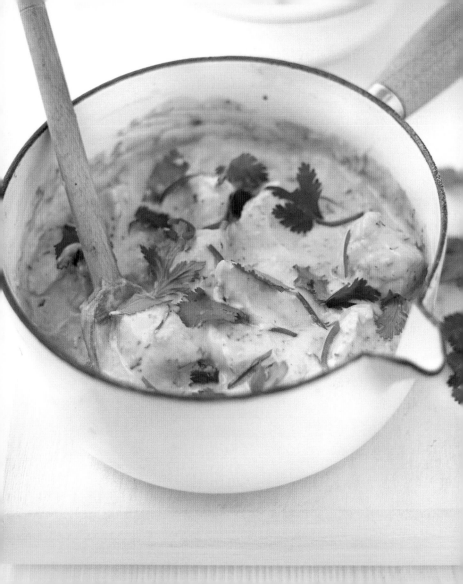

Sticky salmon with Chinese greens

Cook the salmon separately to the stir-fry veg and there's no chance of overcooking either of them.

TAKES 20 MINUTES • SERVES 4

4 skinless salmon fillets (about 150g/5oz each)
3 tbsp oyster sauce
2 tbsp teriyaki sauce
1 tbsp clear honey
1 tbsp oil (a mix of vegetable and sesame)
1 tbsp finely grated ginger
1 garlic clove, finely sliced
1 red chilli, deseeded and finely sliced
500g/1lb 2oz mixed green veg – we used pak choi, sugar snaps and broccoli

1 Heat oven to 200C/180C fan/gas 6. Put the salmon on a baking sheet. Mix the oyster and teriyaki sauces with the honey, then brush a little over the fish. Roast for 8–10 minutes until glazed and just cooked through. Set aside and keep warm.

2 Meanwhile, heat the oil in a wok, then fry the ginger, garlic and chilli for 1 minute. Stir-fry the broccoli or any larger, harder veg for 3 minutes, then add the leafy veg and cook for 1–2 minutes more. Stir in the rest of the sticky sauce, heat through and serve with the fish.

PER SERVING 354 kcals, protein 35g, carbs 10g, fat 20g, sat fat 4g, fibre 2g, sugar 8g, salt 2.81g

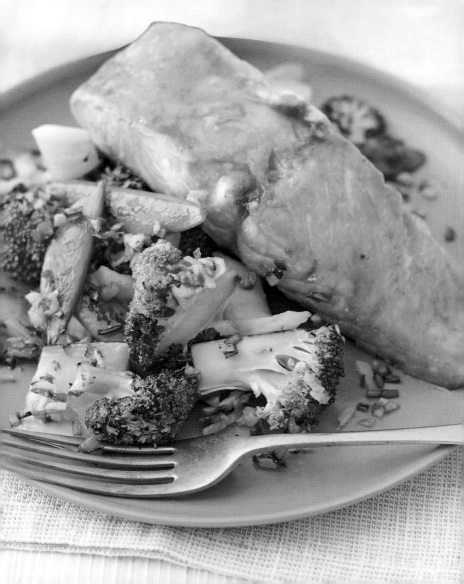

Butternut & broccoli supersalad with mackerel

Brimming with protective antioxidants, this satisfying salad combines ingredients rich in vitamin E.

TAKES 40 MINUTES ● SERVES 2

1 tsp white wine vinegar
1 tsp wholegrain mustard
1 tbsp olive oil
200g/7oz butternut squash (about ½ small squash), peeled, deseeded and cut into 2cm/¾in chunks
85g/3oz green beans, trimmed and halved
140g/5oz long-stemmed broccoli, halved vertically
1 tbsp pumpkin seeds
4 mackerel fillets, bones removed

1 Whisk together the vinegar, mustard, 2 teaspoons of the oil and a little seasoning in a large bowl.

2 Bring a large pan of salted water to the boil and heat the remaining oil in a large frying pan. Add the squash to the frying pan, season and cook, stirring, for 12–15 minutes. Add the beans to the water, cook for 1 minute, then add the broccoli and cook for 3 minutes more. Drain well.

3 Tip the squash into the bowl with the dressing. Add the beans, broccoli and pumpkin seeds, toss well to combine and set aside. Cook the fish in the frying pan, skin-side down, for 2 minutes, then flip over and cook for a further 1–2 minutes until cooked through.

4 Divide the salad between the plates, top with the mackerel and drizzle over any dressing left in the bowl.

PER SERVING 501 kcals, protein 35g, carbs 12g, fat 35g, sat fat 7g, fibre 5g, sugar 7g, salt 0.6g

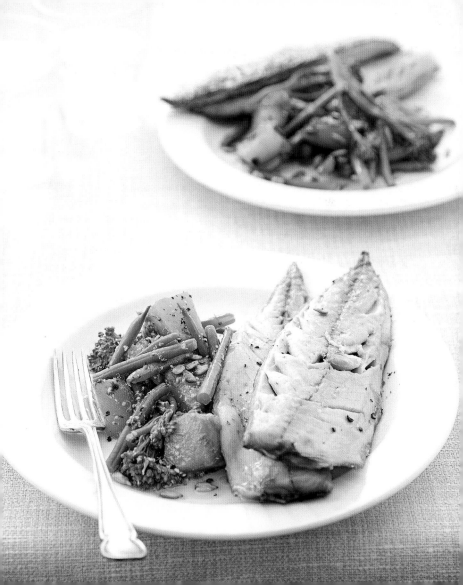

Sticky green stir-fry with beef

Keep the heat high under the pan as you fry the steak – you don't want it to steam and overcook.

TAKES 20 MINUTES • **SERVES 4**

1 tbsp sunflower oil

2 × 200g/7oz sirloin steaks, trimmed of fat and thinly sliced

1 head broccoli, cut into small florets

2 garlic cloves, sliced

300g/10oz sugar snap peas

4 spring onions, thickly sliced

3 pak choi, leaves separated and cut into quarters

4 tbsp hoisin sauce

1 Heat the oil in a large wok or deep frying pan, then sizzle the beef strips for 3–4 minutes until browned. Remove and set aside.

2 Toss the broccoli and garlic into the wok with a splash of water, then fry over a high heat for 4–5 minutes until starting to soften. Add the peas, spring onions and pak choi, stir-fry for another 2–3 minutes, then stir in the hoisin sauce and the beef. Heat through quickly, adding a splash of water if it seems a little dry, and serve straightaway.

PER SERVING 253 kcals, protein 32g, carbs 13g, fat 9g, sat fat 2g, fibre 5g, sugar 10g, salt 0.82g

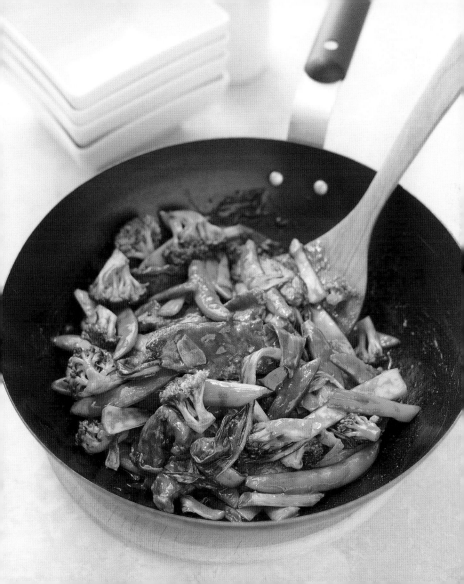

Roast pork with apples & mustard

Tangy apples and hot mustard ensure this dish is packed full of punchy flavours.

TAKES 50 MINUTES • **SERVES 4**

1 tbsp olive oil
3 eating apples
500g/1lb 2oz pork fillet, sliced into
    medallions
200ml/7fl oz reduced-salt chicken
    stock
1 tbsp wholegrain mustard
1 tbsp chopped sage leaves
2 tbsp half-fat crème fraîche
mashed potato, to serve

1 Heat half the oil in a large frying pan. Core and cut the apples into wedges, then cook for about 10 minutes until caramelised and softened. Remove from the pan and set aside. Heat the remaining oil. Fry the pork on each side for 2 minutes.

2 Add the stock and mustard to the pan, then bubble for 5 minutes or until the pork is cooked through. Return the apples to the pan with the sage and cook for 1 minute more.

3 Remove from the heat and stir in the crème fraîche and some seasoning. Serve with mash.

PER SERVING 246 kcals, protein 28g, carbs 12g, fat 10g, sat fat 3g, fibre 2g, sugar 11g, salt 0.39g

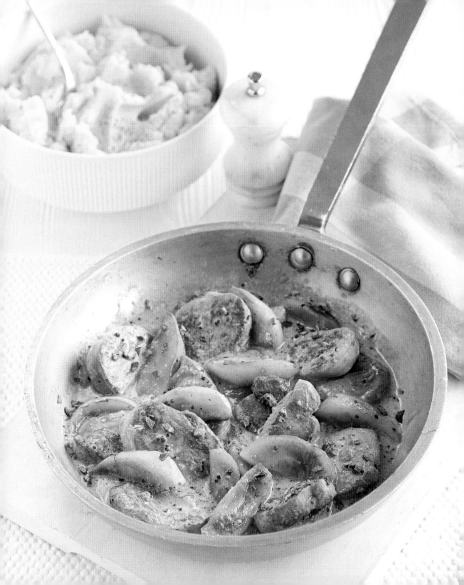

Stuffed-marrow bake

Kids will love this budget-friendly supper just as much as you will.

TAKES 1 HOUR • SERVES 6

1 tbsp olive oil
1 onion, chopped
1 garlic clove, crushed
1 tbsp dried mixed herbs
500g pack minced turkey
2 × 400g cans chopped tomatoes
1 marrow, cut into 4cm/1½in-thick
  slices
4 tbsp very finely chopped almonds
3 tbsp grated Parmesan

1 Heat oven to 200C/180C fan/gas 6. Heat the oil in a large frying pan and cook the onion and garlic with 2 teaspoons of the herbs for 3 minutes until starting to soften. Add the turkey and brown all over, then tip in the tomatoes and cook for 5 minutes more.

2 Scoop out the middle of the marrow and discard (or fry, then freeze for another time – try it mashed with celeriac). Arrange the slices in a baking dish. Spoon the mince into the middle of each marrow slice, then spoon the rest over the top. Cover with foil and bake for 30 minutes.

3 Meanwhile, mix the remaining herbs with the almonds and Parmesan. Remove the marrow from the oven, uncover, and sprinkle over the nut mixture. Return to the oven for 10 minutes more until topping is golden and crisp and the marrow is tender.

PER SERVING 240 kcals, protein 27g, carbs 8g, fat 11g, sat fat 2g, fibre 2g, sugar 7g, salt 0.4g

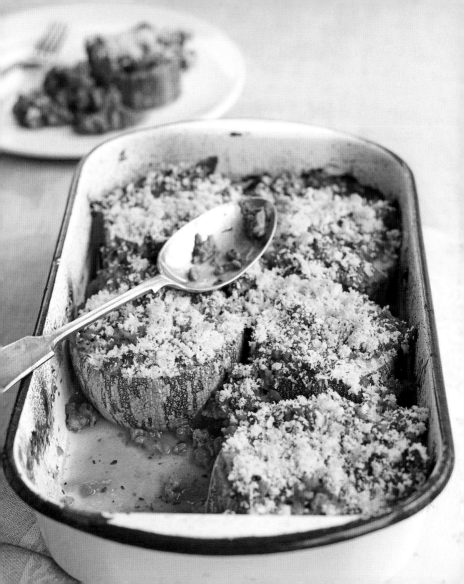

Red Thai meatball curry

If you need a short cut, you can save yourself 10 minutes of rolling time if you buy ready-made meatballs from the supermarket.

TAKES 40 MINUTES • SERVES 4

500g pack lean minced beef (10% fat)
2 red chillies, 1 chopped, 1 sliced
thumb-size piece ginger, grated
1 beaten egg
1 tbsp sunflower or vegetable oil
1–1½ tbsp Thai red curry paste
  (depending on how spicy you like it)
400ml can reduced-fat coconut milk
225g can bamboo shoots, drained
140g/5oz fine green beans, trimmed
juice 1 lime, plus extra wedges to
  squeeze over
20g pack basil leaves

1 Put the mince into a large bowl with the chopped chilli, ginger and egg, then season generously. Mix well with your hands, then shape into 20 meatballs. The meatballs can be made and chilled up to a day ahead.

2 Heat the oil in a large non-stick frying pan, then brown the meatballs for 5 minutes. Tip on to a plate. Add the curry paste to the pan, fry for 1 minute, then pour in the coconut milk and half a can of water. Bring back to the boil and stir to make a smooth sauce.

3 Return the meatballs to the pan with the bamboo shoots and beans. Simmer for 5 minutes until the beans are just tender and meatballs cooked through. To serve, season the sauce with some salt and pepper and the lime juice, then tear in the basil leaves. Scatter with the sliced chilli and serve with the lime wedges for squeezing over.

PER SERVING 371 kcals, protein 31g, carbs 4g, fat 26g, sat fat 13g, fibre 2g, sugar 2g, salt 0.79g

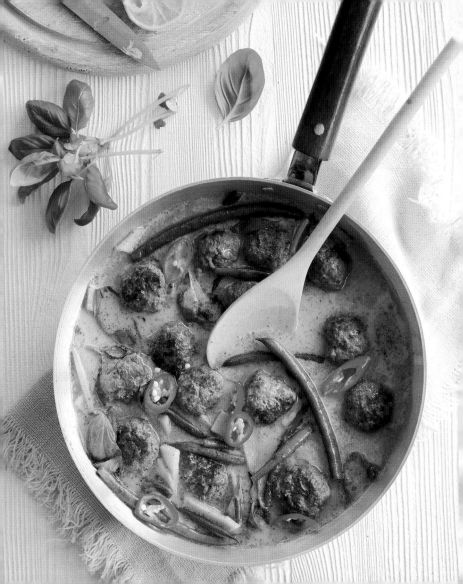

Satay pork with crunchy apple salad

This healthy meal is simple to prepare and packed with flavour, and it is very easily halved if there are just two of you.

TAKES 20 MINUTES • SERVES 4

3 tbsp crunchy peanut butter
3 tbsp sweet chilli sauce
4 lean pork steaks
juice 2 limes
1 tsp Thai fish sauce
pinch sugar
2 apples, cored and thinly sliced
small pack coriander, leaves roughly torn
½ small pack mint, leaves roughly torn

1 Heat the grill. Mix the peanut butter and sweet chilli sauce together, then season with freshly ground black pepper (the peanut butter is salty enough). Arrange the pork on a baking sheet, brush the tops with half the nutty mixture, then grill for 3 minutes. Carefully turn the pork steaks over, brush with the remaining mixture, then grill for 3–4 minutes more until just cooked through.

2 Meanwhile, make the salad by mixing the lime juice, fish sauce and sugar in a bowl. Stir in the apple slices so they are well coated in the dressing, then toss with the coriander and mint. Serve the crunchy apple salad alongside the pork steaks.

PER SERVING 310 kcals, protein 36g, carbs 15g, fat 12g, sat fat 3g, fibre 2g, sugar 15g, salt 1.08g

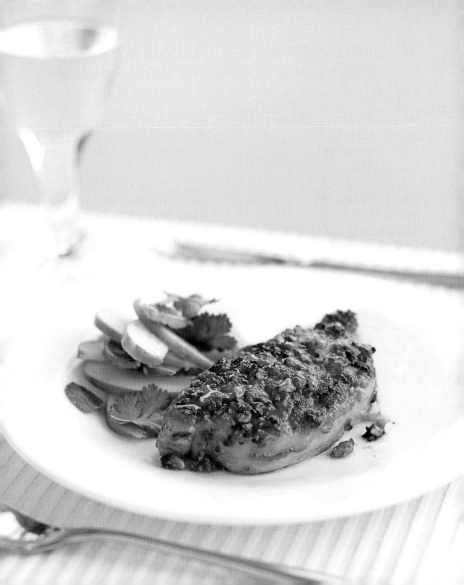

Griddled salmon with spring-onion dressing

This easy spring-onion dressing is also great with just about any barbecued meat or poultry.

TAKES 30 MINUTES • SERVES 4

4 skin-on salmon fillets
olive oil, for brushing
lemon wedges and a big bowl of
   watercress salad, to serve

FOR THE DRESSING

1 bunch spring onions
large handful flat-leaf parsley leaves,
   chopped
½ red chilli, finely chopped (seeds in or
   out – up to you)
4 tbsp olive oil
juice ½ lemon
1 tbsp sherry vinegar

1 To make the dressing, chop the spring onions as finely as possible without turning them to mush. Tip into a bowl with the parsley and chilli. Drizzle in the oil, stirring until the ingredients are just bound, then stir in the lemon juice and vinegar. Season with salt and set aside.

2 Heat the griddle until hot and brush the salmon with a little oil. Cook the salmon fillets for 4 minutes on each side until just cooked through. Serve on a platter with the dressing, lemon wedges for squeezing over and a bowl of watercress salad for everyone to help themselves to.

PER SERVING 367 kcals, protein 29g, carbs 1g, fat 28g, sat fat 5g, fibre 1g, sugar 1g, salt 0.17g

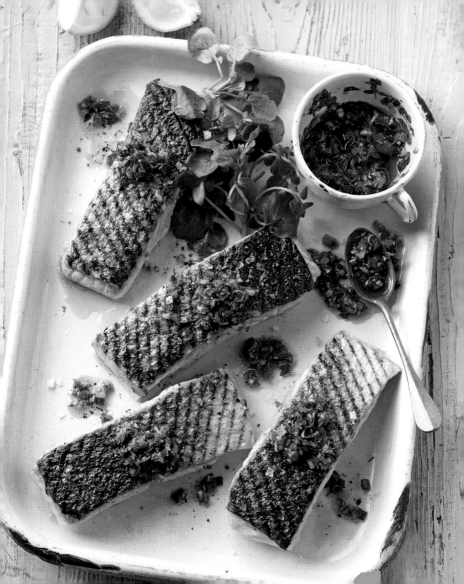

Gammon & cauliflower-cheese grills

Mixing crème fraîche with cheese makes an easy cheese sauce that can be used with lots of different vegetables, or for baking with chicken breasts.

TAKES 30 MINUTES • SERVES 4

4 small raw gammon steaks
1 large cauliflower, cut into florets
1 tbsp wholegrain mustard
100ml/3fl oz half-fat crème fraîche
85g/3oz Cheddar, grated

1 Heat the grill to high. Snip the sides of the gammon steaks with kitchen scissors so they don't curl up too much when they cook. Put the gammon on to a baking sheet, then grill on one side for about 10 minutes until the fat is crisp.

2 Meanwhile, cook the cauliflower in boiling water for 5 minutes until tender. Drain and tip into a bowl with the mustard, crème fraîche and two-thirds of the cheese, and give it all a good mix.

3 When the gammon is crisp, flip it over and cook on the other side for about 10 minutes. Spoon the cauliflower mix over the gammon, sprinkle with cheese, then grill for 5 minutes until bubbling and golden.

PER SERVING 420 kcals, protein 36g, carbs 9g, fat 27g, sat fat 13g, fibre 4g, sugar 7g, salt 3.58g

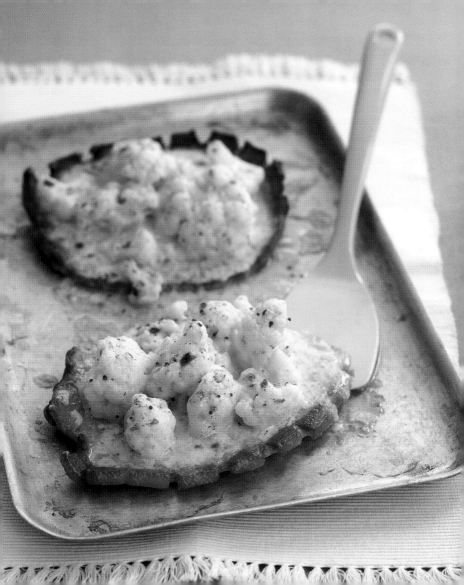

Spicy baby aubergine stew with coriander & mint

You'll find baby aubergines in Middle Eastern and Asian stores, and also in some larger supermarkets.

TAKES 55 MINUTES • **SERVES 4**

2 tbsp olive oil
1 red onion, sliced
4 garlic cloves, smashed
2 red chillies, deseeded and sliced, or
 2–3 dried red chillies, left whole
2 tsp coriander seeds, toasted and
 crushed
2 tsp cumin seeds, toasted and
 crushed
16 baby aubergines, left whole with
 stalk intact
2 × 400g cans chopped tomatoes
1 tsp sugar
bunch mint, roughly chopped
bunch coriander, roughly chopped
natural yogurt, to serve

1 Heat the oil in a heavy-based pan, add the onion and garlic, and cook until they begin to colour. Add the chillies, coriander and cumin seeds. When the seeds give off a nutty aroma, toss in the whole aubergines, coating them in the onion and spices.
2 Tip in the tomatoes and sugar, cover and gently cook for 40 minutes, until the aubergines are tender.
3 Season the sauce and toss in half the mint and coriander. Cover and simmer for 2 minutes. Sprinkle over the remaining herbs and serve with yogurt.

PER SERVING 135 kcals, protein 5g, carbs 14g, fat 7g, sat fat 1g, fibre 6g, sugar 12g, salt 0.31g

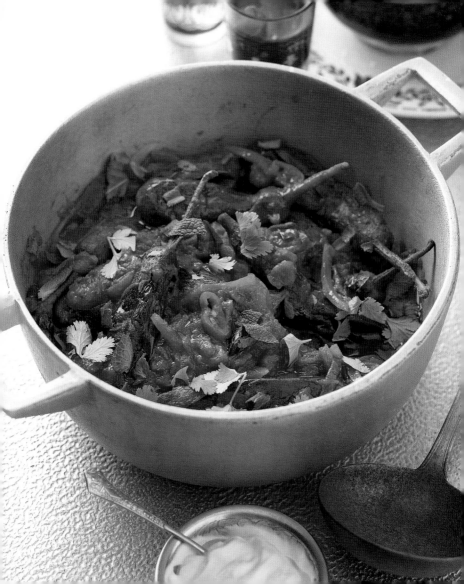

Sweet & spicy wings with summer slaw

A great option for a midweek meal that won't break the bank; chicken wings are good fun, but really inexpensive.

TAKES 1 HOUR • SERVES 4

4 tbsp curry paste (we used tikka)
3 tbsp mango chutney
1kg/2lb 4oz chicken wings
200g bag radishes, sliced
1 cucumber, halved lengthways and
    sliced
small bunch mint, roughly chopped
juice 1 lemon

1 Heat oven to 200C/180C fan/gas 6. In a large bowl, mix the curry paste with 2 tablespoons of the mango chutney and some seasoning. Tip in the wings and toss to combine so they are well coated. Lay the wings in a single layer on a large baking sheet or two smaller ones. Roast for 40–45 minutes until cooked through and golden (or barbecue, turning, until cooked through).

2 Meanwhile, mix the radishes and cucumber with the mint, remaining mango chutney and the lemon juice. Transfer to a serving bowl. Pile the wings on a big plate and serve with the summer slaw.

PER SERVING 591 kcals, protein 48g, carbs 11g, fat 39g, sat fat 12g, fibre 2g, sugar 8g, salt 1.67g

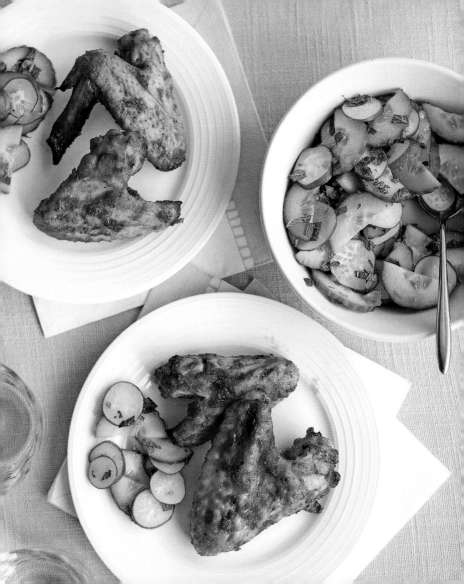

Prosciutto & pesto fish gratin

Fancy this with chicken instead? Wrap the prosciutto around 4 skinless chicken breasts then follow as below, but bake for 20–25 minutes until the chicken is cooked.

TAKES 20 MINUTES • SERVES 4

4 chunky white fish fillets
4 slices prosciutto
200g pot crème fraîche
3 tbsp basil pesto
25g/1oz Parmesan, finely grated
1 tbsp pine nuts

1 Heat oven to 200C/180C fan/gas 6. Season the fish all over, then wrap each fillet in a slice of prosciutto. Put into a large baking dish. Dot the crème fraîche among the fillets and over the exposed ends of the fish. Dot the pesto around the fish, too. Scatter with the cheese.
2 Bake the fish for 15–20 minutes, adding the pine nuts halfway through, until the crème fraîche has made a sauce around the fish, and the cheese and ham are turning golden.

PER SERVING 406 kcals, protein 34g, carbs 2g, fat 29g, sat fat 16g, fibre none, sugar 1g, salt 0.82g

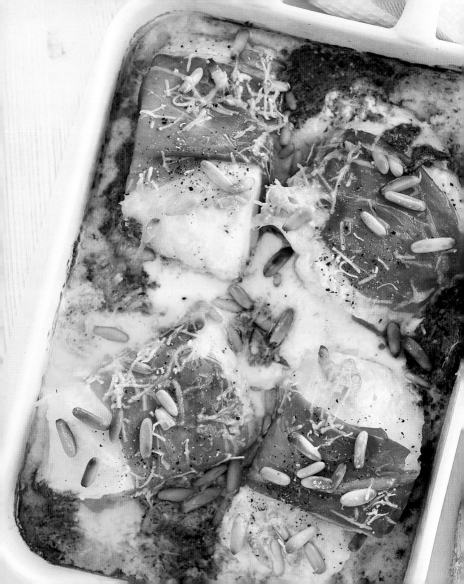

Mediterranean vegetables with lamb

If you like ratatouille you'll really enjoy this one-pot version with lots of lovely lamb.

TAKES 45 MINUTES ● SERVES 4

1 tbsp olive oil

250g/9oz lean lamb fillet, trimmed of any fat and thinly sliced

140g/5oz shallots, halved

2 large courgettes, cut into chunks

½ tsp each ground cumin, paprika and ground coriander

1 red, 1 yellow and 1 green pepper, deseeded and cut into chunks

1 garlic clove, sliced

150ml/¼ pint vegetable stock

250g/9oz cherry tomatoes

handful coriander leaves, roughly chopped

1 Heat the oil in a large heavy-based pan with a lid. Cook the lamb and shallots over a high heat for 2–3 minutes until golden. Add the courgettes and stir-fry for 3–4 minutes until beginning to soften.

2 Add the spices and toss well, then add the peppers and garlic. Reduce the heat and cook over a moderate heat for 4–5 minutes until they start to soften.

3 Pour in the stock and stir to coat. Add the tomatoes, season, then cover with a lid and simmer for 15 minutes, stirring occasionally until the veg are tender. Stir through the coriander to serve.

PER SERVING 192 kcals, protein 17g, carbs 11g, fat 9g, sat fat 3g, fibre 4g, sugar 10g, salt 0.25g

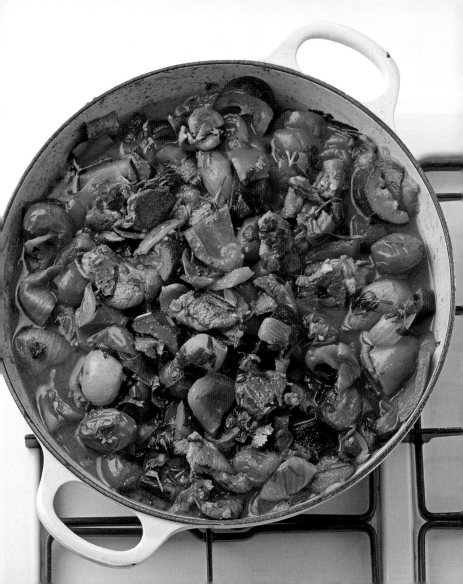

Baked fish with mint & mango relish

Why not serve this with an Indian-style green salad? Just mix together diced cucumber, sliced spring onions, mixed salad leaves, coriander and lime juice.

TAKES 30 MINUTES ● SERVES 4

4 × 150g thick line-caught skinless cod fillets
1 green chilli, finely chopped (seeds in or out, it's up to you)
1 small ripe mango, finely diced
1 tsp ground cumin
½ finger-length piece ginger, grated
large handful mint leaves, shredded
1 tbsp mango chutney
juice ½ lime
85g/3oz blanched almonds
1 tsp garam masala
½ tsp turmeric powder
1 tbsp olive oil
green salad, to serve

1 Heat oven to 200C/180C fan/gas 6 and put the fish fillets in a roasting tin. Combine the chopped chilli, mango, cumin, ginger, mint, mango chutney and lime juice. Spoon a quarter of the relish on top of each fillet and pat it down into an even layer with your fingers.

2 Put the almonds in a food processor with the garam masala and turmeric, and whizz to fine crumbs. Add the olive oil and give the processor one final pulse to mix everything together.

3 Spoon the crumbs over the relish-topped fillets. Cover the tin with foil and bake for 10 minutes. Remove the foil and continue cooking for another 5 minutes until the fish flakes easily and the crumbs have crisped on top. Serve with a green salad.

PER SERVING 321 kcals, protein 33g, carbs 12g, fat 16g, sat fat 2g, fibre 2g, sugar 10g, salt 0.4g

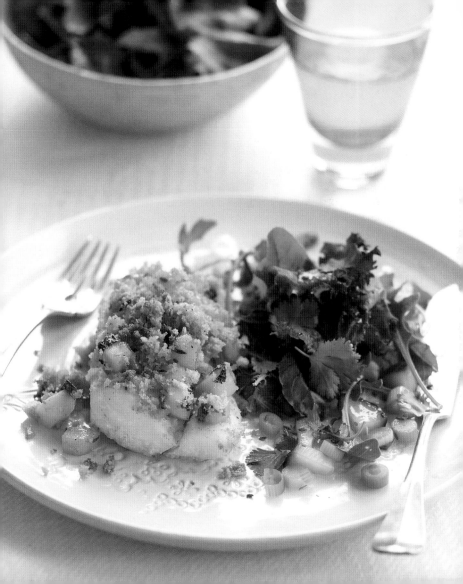

Roasted beets with watercress & horseradish-apple sauce

Serve with grilled salmon, beef steaks or pork chops. This recipe is easily halved.

TAKES 2 HOURS 20 MINUTES

● **SERVES 8**

1kg/2lb 4oz raw unpeeled beetroot
2 apples, peeled and chopped
1 tbsp sugar
2 tbsp cider vinegar or red wine vinegar
6 tbsp freshly grated horseradish
4 tbsp soured cream
2 bunches watercress

1 Heat oven to 200C/180C fan/gas 6. If your beetroot comes with leafy tops, cut them down, making sure you leave about a 3cm/1¼in stalk intact. Wrap them individually in foil and roast until tender when pierced – about 1–2 hours (depending on their size). Cool in the foil before peeling then set aside.

2 To make the sauce, heat a small frying pan with a lid, then toss in the apples with the sugar and 1 tablespoon water. Cover and cook until the apples are soft and mushy. Remove from the heat, add the vinegar and blitz to a purée using a stick blender or food processor. Stir in the horseradish and soured cream, and season with some salt to taste.

3 To serve, cut the beetroot into wedges, put in a bowl and mix with the sauce. Serve on a bed of watercress.

PER SERVING 87 kcals, protein 3g, carbs 15g, fat 2g, sat fat 1g, fibre 4g, sugar 14g, salt 0.23g

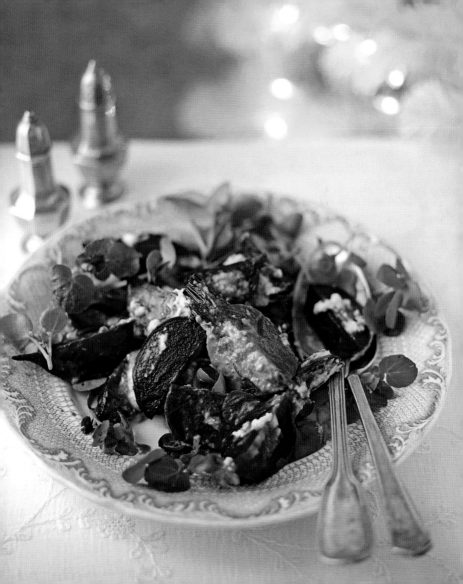

Root vegetable & mustard mash

Make the most of cheap and tasty seasonal root vegetables, and you won't even miss the spuds!

TAKES 35 MINUTES • SERVES 8

1 swede, peeled and cut into
  small chunks
1 celeriac, peeled and cut into
  small chunks
6 carrots, peeled and cut into
  small chunks
50g/2oz butter
3 tbsp extra virgin olive oil
2 tbsp wholegrain mustard

1 Put the veg in a large pan of salted water. Bring to the boil and cook for 15 minutes until tender.
2 Drain well, then mash adding the butter, oil and mustard. Season generously. Mix together until the butter has melted, and serve piping hot.

PER SERVING 152 kcals, protein 2g, carbs 13g, fat 11g, sat fat 4g, fibre 7g, sugar 12g, salt 0.51g

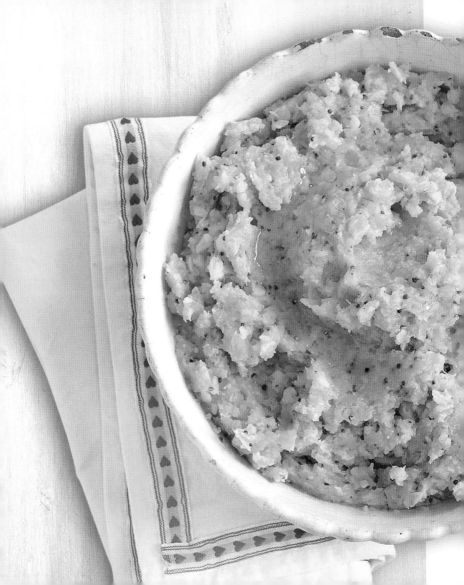

Broccoli with sautéed bacon & onions

A great way to liven up broccoli – serve with chicken breasts simply roasted with olive oil, salt and pepper.

TAKES 20 MINUTES ● **SERVES 4**

300g/10oz long-stemmed broccoli,
  ends trimmed
1 tsp olive oil
1 onion, finely chopped
140g/5oz streaky bacon, chopped
2 garlic cloves, finely chopped

1 Cook the broccoli for 3 minutes in boiling salted water. Drain, run under cold water until completely cooled, then set aside.

2 Heat the oil in a large frying pan, add the onion and bacon, and cook on a medium heat for about 10 minutes, adding the garlic halfway through, until the bacon is crisp and the onions are soft and golden.

3 Add the broccoli to the pan, then toss through to coat in the oil. Cook for a couple more minutes until the broccoli is completely heated through. Season with some freshly ground black pepper; then serve immediately.

PER SERVING 126 kcals, protein 8g, carbs 5g, fat 9g, sat fat 3g, fibre 3g, sugar 3g, salt 1.09g

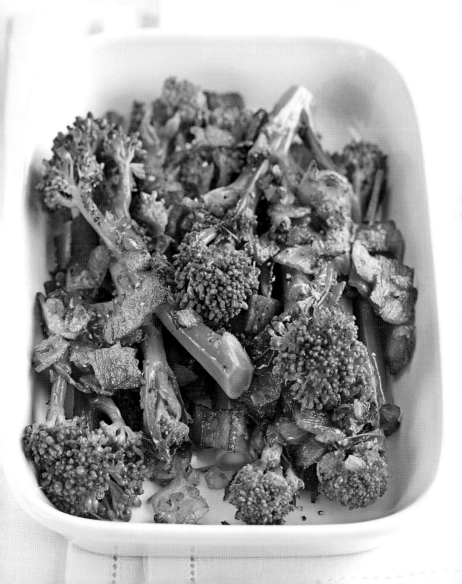

Green beans with shallots, garlic & almonds

These beans work alongside any Italian or French dishes, or even as part of a Sunday roast.

TAKES 15 MINUTES • SERVES 4

300g/10oz green beans, trimmed
2 tbsp olive oil
2 shallots, thinly sliced
3 garlic cloves, thinly sliced
squeeze lemon juice
2 tbsp toasted flaked almonds

1 Cook the green beans in boiling salted water until tender, then drain and cool under running water. Set aside.

2 Put the olive oil, shallots, garlic and some salt in a frying pan, then cook gently for about 8 minutes until soft but not brown. Tip in the beans and a grind of black pepper, toss well, then warm through.

3 Finish with a squeeze of lemon and a scattering of the toasted flaked almonds.

PER SERVING 47 kcals, protein 3g, carbs 3g, fat 3g, sat fat none, fibre 2g, sugar 2g, salt none

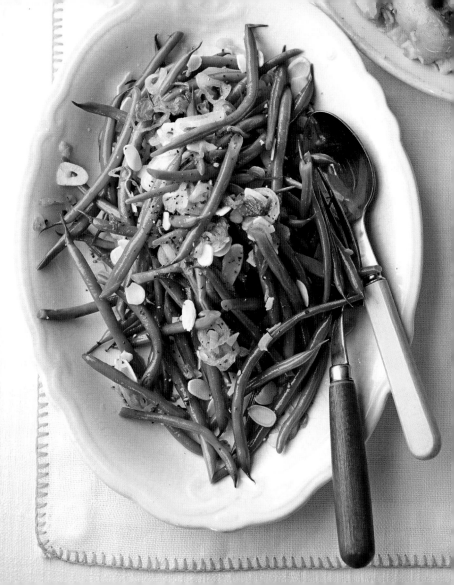

Roast tomatoes

Tomatoes take on an intensely deep flavour after roasting and can be used to perk up a main course.

TAKES 1 HOUR 10 MINUTES
- **SERVES 4**

10 large vine tomatoes, halved
4 garlic cloves, sliced
½ bunch thyme
3 tbsp balsamic vinegar
2 tbsp olive oil

1 Heat oven to 160C/140C fan/gas 3. Put the tomatoes on a baking sheet with the garlic and thyme, drizzle over the balsamic vinegar and olive oil, add some seasoning and roast for 1 hour.

2 Remove from the oven and allow to cool to room temperature before eating.

PER SERVING 115 kcals, protein 3g, carbs 12g, fat 7g, sat fat 1g, fibre 3g, sugar 11g, salt 0.07g

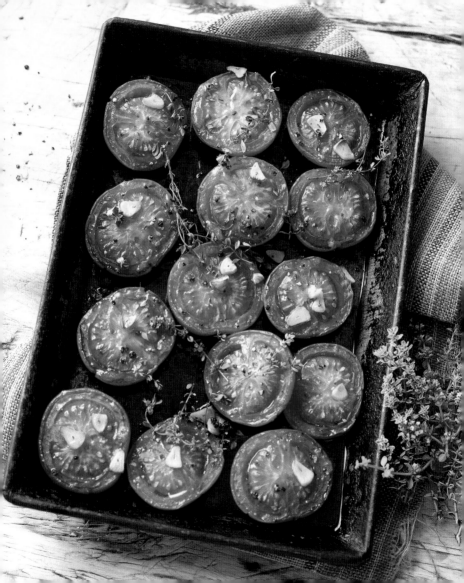

Creamed spinach

Everyone will enjoy this rich and creamy side dish, and it's pretty versatile, too – it's great with white fish, pork, beef steaks or chicken.

TAKES 25 MINUTES • SERVES 8

25g/1oz butter
1 small onion, finely chopped
2 tbsp plain flour
200ml/7fl oz full-fat milk
2 × 200g bags spinach leaves
100ml/3½fl oz single cream
grating fresh nutmeg

1 Heat the butter in a pan, then add the onion and cook for 5 minutes until softened. Stir in the flour and cook for 2 minutes, then slowly start to whisk in the milk. When it has all been incorporated, gently cook for 5 minutes until the sauce has thickened.

2 Meanwhile, put the spinach in a large colander. Pour over a kettle full of boiling water until the leaves have wilted (you may have to do this twice). Put the spinach in a clean dishcloth, squeeze out any excess liquid, then roughly chop.

3 Stir the spinach into the sauce with the cream, gently heat, then finely grate over some nutmeg and season well to serve.

PER SERVING 83 kcals, protein 3g, carbs 5g, fat 6g, sat fat 4g, fibre 1g, sugar 3g, salt 0.26g

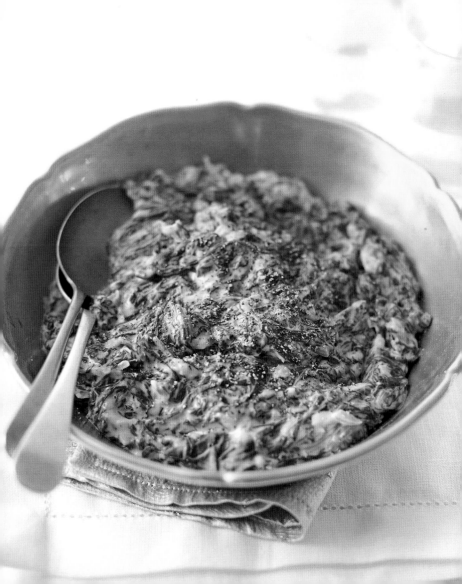

Sticky carrots with thyme & honey

Try Chantenay carrots for this recipe if you can find them or, failing that, use sweet baby carrots with their leafy tops.

TAKES 35 MINUTES • SERVES 8

1kg/2lb 4oz Chantenay carrots,
    unpeeled, larger ones halved
25g/1oz butter
few thyme sprigs
1 tbsp honey

1 Tip the carrots into a deep frying pan with the butter, thyme and honey. Cook for 5 minutes until starting to brown.
2 Pour in 250ml/9fl oz water, bring to the boil and cook until the water has evaporated and the carrots are tender. Turn down the heat and cook the carrots slowly, stirring, until glazed.

PER SERVING 73 kcals, protein 1g, carbs 11g, fat 3g, sat fat 2g, fibre 3g, sugar 11g, salt 0.12g

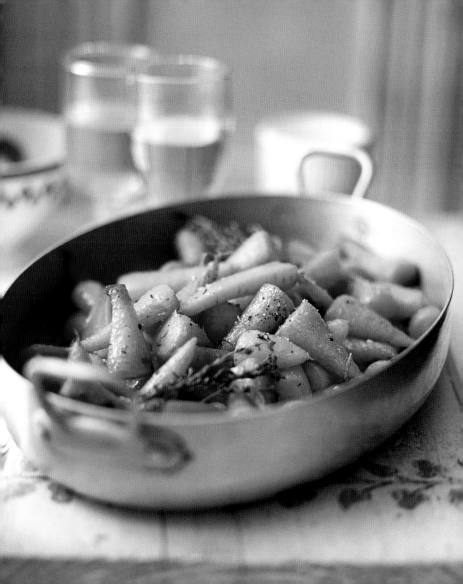

Roasted cauliflower with garlic, bay & lemon

If you don't fancy garlic, roast the cauliflower with a little deseeded and chopped red chilli or a sprinkle of smoked paprika or cumin seeds.

TAKES 30 MINUTES • SERVES 8

2 heads cauliflower, cut into even bite-sized pieces
1 garlic bulb, split into cloves, unpeeled
6 bay leaves, stalks removed, finely chopped
4 tbsp olive oil
zest and juice 1 lemon

1 Heat oven to 200C/180C fan/gas 6. Put the cauliflower, garlic and bay leaves in a large bowl, toss with the oil, lemon zest and juice, and season generously.
2 Spread evenly on to a baking sheet (use two if you need to). Roast for 20 minutes, turning halfway through, until al dente and caramelised.

PER SERVING 96 kcals, protein 5g, carbs 5g, fat 7g, sat fat 1g, fibre 2g, sugar 3g, salt 0.03g

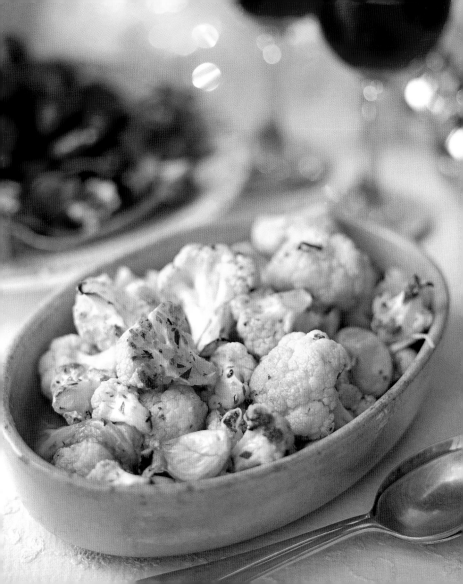

Sprouts with chestnuts & bacon

This combination of sprouts with salty bacon and earthy chestnuts is a winner.

TAKES 15 MINUTES ● SERVES 8

1.25kg/2lb 12oz Brussels sprouts, trimmed (or if using pre-trimmed, buy 1kg/2lb 4oz)

6 rashers streaky smoked bacon, cut into bite-sized pieces

140g/5oz vacuum-packed chestnuts, halved

50g/2oz butter

1 Bring a large pan of salted water to the boil, then tip in the sprouts. Once back to the boil, cook for 5 minutes. Drain, run under the cold tap until cold, then drain again.

2 Heat a large frying pan, add the bacon and gently fry for 10 minutes until crisp and golden. Tip out of the pan, leaving the fat behind, then add the chestnuts and fry over a high heat for about 5 minutes until tinged. Tip out of the pan.

3 Add the sprouts to the pan with a splash of water, then cover and finish cooking over a medium heat for about 5 minutes, stirring now and again, until just tender. Uncover, turn up the heat, then add most of the butter and sauté the sprouts for 2 minutes more. Tip in the bacon and chestnuts, season generously, then serve with the last knob of butter on top.

PER SERVING 183 kcals, protein 8g, carbs 12g, fat 12g, sat fat 5g, fibre 7g, sugar 6g, salt 0.61g

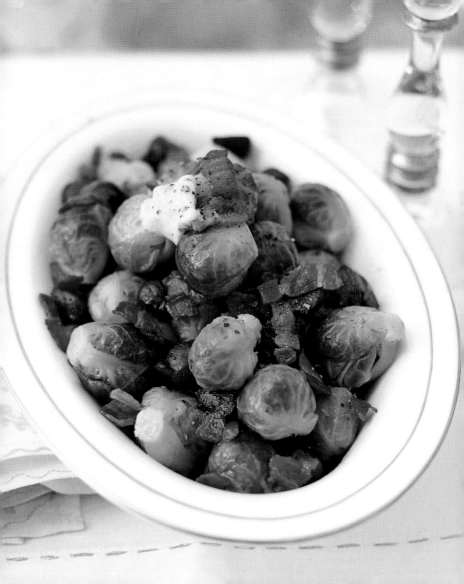

Broad beans with peas & mint butter

Broad beans and peas are in season in the spring, but during the rest of the year frozen ones will be fine.

TAKES 45 MINUTES • SERVES 8

50g/2oz butter
1 bunch spring onions, chopped
700g/1lb 9oz podded broad beans
4 tbsp chicken stock or water
500g/1lb 2oz podded peas
handful mint leaves

1 Heat half the butter in a frying pan and fry the onions until soft. Add the beans and stir, then pour in the stock or water, bring to the boil, cover and cook for 5 minutes.
2 Add the peas and some seasoning, and cook for 5 minutes until tender. Stir in the mint and remaining butter.

PER SERVING 97 kcals, protein 5g, carbs 7g, fat 6g, sat fat 4g, fibre 4g, sugar 2g, salt 0.10g

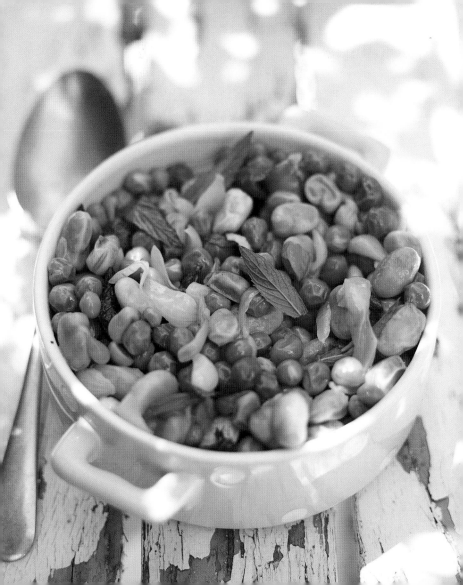

Red cabbage with port & cranberries

If you like braised red cabbage, you'll love this modern version of this popular dish. Here the red cabbage is cooked with port and sharp cranberries.

TAKES 1 HOUR 10 MINUTES
- **SERVES 8**

3 tbsp olive oil
2 large onions, halved and thinly sliced
1 tsp ground cloves
1 medium red cabbage, quartered, cored and thinly sliced
200ml/7fl oz vegetable stock
3 tbsp port
3 tbsp brown sugar
100g/4oz fresh or frozen cranberries

1 Heat the oil in a large pan, then add the onions and fry, stirring every now and then, for about 10 minutes, until they start to caramelise. Stir in the cloves, then add the cabbage and continue cooking, stirring more frequently this time, until the cabbage starts to soften.

2 Pour in the stock, add the port and sugar, then cover, and cook for 10 minutes.

3 Stir in the cranberries and cook for 10 minutes more.

PER SERVING 110 kcals, protein 2g, carbs 14g, fat 5g, sat fat 1g, fibre 5g, sugar 13g, salt 0.1g

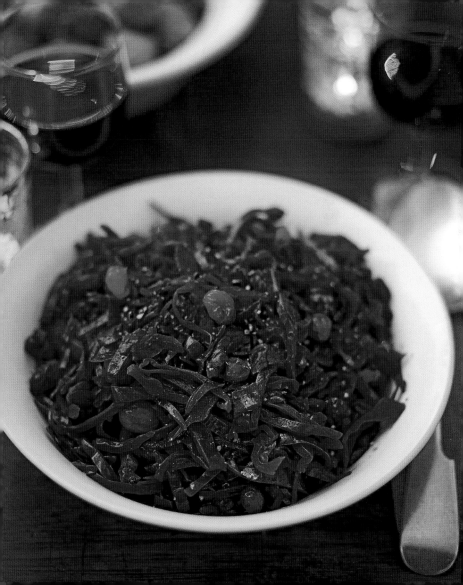

Griddled aubergine with sesame dressing

Tahini paste is like the sesame-seed version of peanut butter and has a lovely intense flavour. Use up the rest of the jar to make your own houmous.

TAKES 30 MINUTES • SERVES 6

2 large aubergines, cut into 2cm/¾in
    slices
2 tbsp olive oil
250g/9oz full-fat Greek yogurt
3 tbsp tahini paste
1 large garlic clove, crushed
juice 1 lemon
handful chopped coriander, parsley
    and mint, plus extra leaves to garnish

1 Brush each aubergine slice with some oil, then season. Heat a griddle pan or barbecue and, when hot, cook the aubergine slices for 2–3 minutes on each side until golden brown and tender.
2 Mix the yogurt with the tahini, garlic, lemon juice and herbs to make a dressing, then season. Top the aubergines with the dressing and scatter over the extra herb leaves to serve.

PER SERVING 194 kcals, protein 7g, carbs 6g, fat 16g, sat fat 5g, fibre 7g, sugar 6g, salt 0.1g

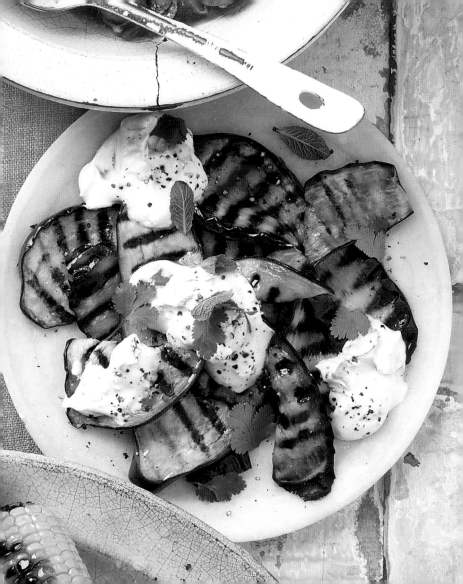

Spring greens with lemon dressing

Add a big bowl of these vibrant greens to a leg of lamb or roast chicken, and your meal is complete!

TAKES 15 MINUTES • SERVES 6–8

250g/9oz broccoli, thicker stalks halved
400g/14oz spring greens, thick stalks
  removed and shredded

FOR THE DRESSING

2 garlic cloves, crushed
zest and juice 1 lemon
2 tbsp olive oil

1 To make the dressing, mix the garlic, lemon juice and zest, olive oil and some seasoning together in a small bowl.
2 Bring a large pan of water to the boil, then add the broccoli and greens, and cook for about 5 minutes until tender. Drain well, then toss through the dressing and serve.

PER SERVING (6) 53 kcals, protein 3g, carbs 2g, fat 4g, sat fat 1g, fibre 3g, sugar 2g, salt none

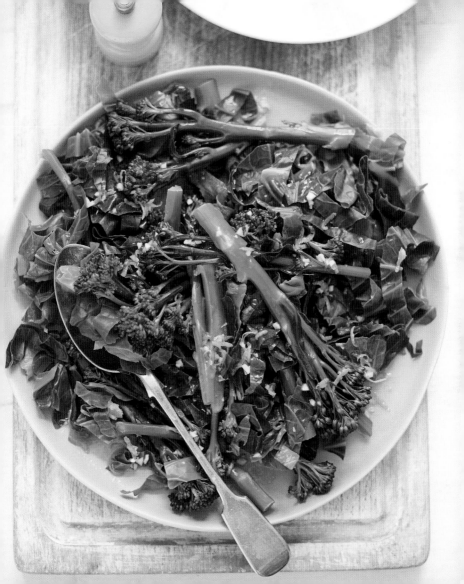

Tomato & onion salad

This salad really is only worth making in the summer when tomatoes are at their sweetest and most flavourful.

TAKES 15 MINUTES • SERVES 8

1kg/2lb 4oz mixed tomatoes (some large, some cherry)
1 red onion, finely chopped
2 tbsp wholegrain mustard
2 tbsp sherry vinegar
2 tbsp clear honey

1 Wash the tomatoes, then cut them all to roughly the same size – halve the cherry tomatoes and chunkily dice or wedge the bigger ones. Stir in the red onion.

2 Whisk together the wholegrain mustard, sherry vinegar and honey with some seasoning. Stir the dressing through the tomatoes and onion up to 2 hours ahead of serving to allow the flavours to combine.

PER SERVING 53 kcals, protein 1g, carbs 9g, fat 1g, sat fat none, fibre 2g, sugar 9g, salt 0.2g

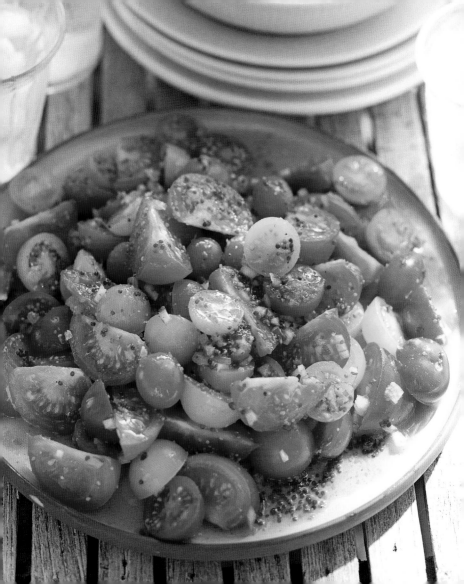

Greek salad

This serves four as a side dish, but is easily doubled to become a main course instead.

TAKES 15 MINUTES ● SERVES 4

4 large vine tomatoes, cut into irregular
  wedges
1 cucumber, peeled, deseeded, then
  roughly chopped
½ red onion, thinly sliced
16 Kalamata olives
1 tsp dried oregano
85g/3oz feta, cut into chunks (barrel-
  matured feta is the best)
4 tbsp Greek extra virgin olive oil

1 Put all of the ingredients in a large
bowl, lightly season, then mix together
well. Serve with lamb – kebabs, chops or
a whole roasted leg on Sundays.

PER SERVING 270 kcals, protein 9g, carbs 8g,
fat 24g, sat fat 6g, fibre 3g, sugar 7g, salt 2.64g

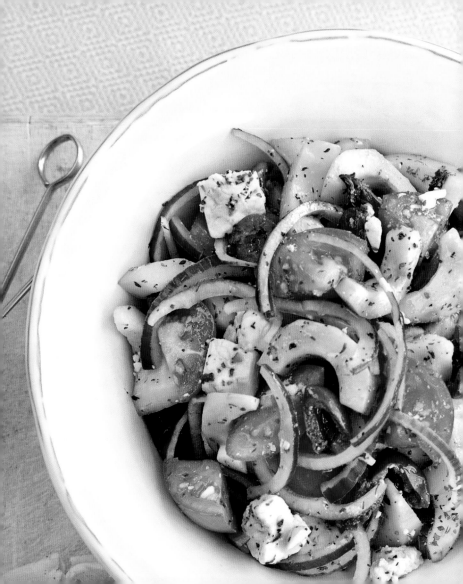

Savoy cabbage with almonds

Green cabbage can be pretty boring, but this recipe is anything but.

TAKES 25 MINUTES • SERVES 8

1 Savoy cabbage, finely sliced
25g/1oz butter
1 tbsp olive oil
1 garlic clove, sliced
1 rosemary sprig, leaves finely chopped
100g/4oz blanched almonds

1 Steam the cabbage or microwave until just cooked.
2 Melt the butter with the oil in a large frying pan or wok, then add the garlic, rosemary and almonds. Cook, stirring the almonds for about 2 minutes or until they start to brown. Tip on to a plate.
3 Add the cabbage to the pan, stir in the leftover buttery juices, then return the almond mixture to the pan. Season well and tip into a serving dish.

PER SERVING 139 kcals, protein 5g, carbs 5g, fat 11g, sat fat 2g, fibre 4g, sugar 4g, salt 0.05g

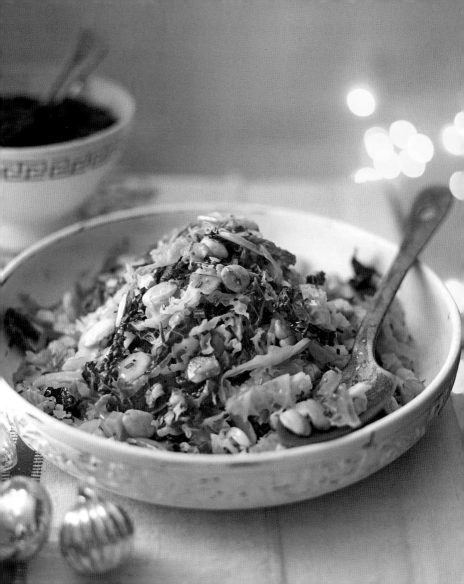

Winter cobb salad

This is the salad for people who don't think they like salad! Full of lots of yummy things to keep every mouthful interesting.

TAKES 25 MINUTES • SERVES 4

6 rashers smoked streaky bacon
2 Little Gem lettuces, chopped
4 celery sticks, chopped
1 roasted chicken breast and leg,
    skinned and shredded
75g/2½oz blue cheese, crumbled
2 hard-boiled eggs, halved

FOR THE DRESSING

4 tbsp olive oil
2 tbsp white wine vinegar
1 tbsp Dijon mustard
1–2 tsp clear honey
2 spring onions, finely sliced

1 Fry the bacon until crisp and cooked through, then very roughly chop and set aside.

2 To make the dressing, mix the olive oil, vinegar, mustard and honey with some seasoning. Stir in the spring onions.

3 Use the chopped lettuce and celery as a base, then arrange the bacon, chicken, blue cheese and hard-boiled eggs on top, and drizzle over the dressing to serve.

PER SERVING 417 kcals, protein 40g, carbs 2g, fat 28g, sat fat 9g, fibre 1g, sugar 2g, salt 2.29g

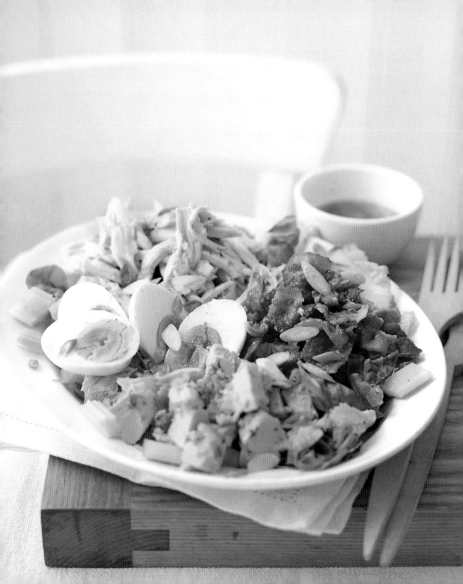

Preserved-lemon & tomato salad with feta

Light and crunchy, tart and fruity, this simple Moroccan salad is deliciously refreshing. Preserved lemons are tangy, but only use the rind – remove the pith and seeds.

TAKES 15 MINUTES • SERVES 4

4 large tomatoes, deseeded
    and cut into thick strips
1 large red onion, thinly sliced
1 preserved lemon, pulp removed
    and rind cut into thin strips
200g pack feta cheese
2 tbsp olive oil
juice ½ lemon
small bunch flat-leaf parsley, finely
    shredded
small bunch mint, leaves finely
    shredded

1 Put the tomatoes, onion and lemon in a shallow bowl or on a platter. Crumble the feta over, drizzle with oil and lemon juice, and scatter over the herbs.
2 Toss gently just before serving.

PER SERVING 215 kcals, protein 10g, carbs 9g, fat 16g, sat fat 7g, fibre 2g, sugar 7g, salt 1.49g

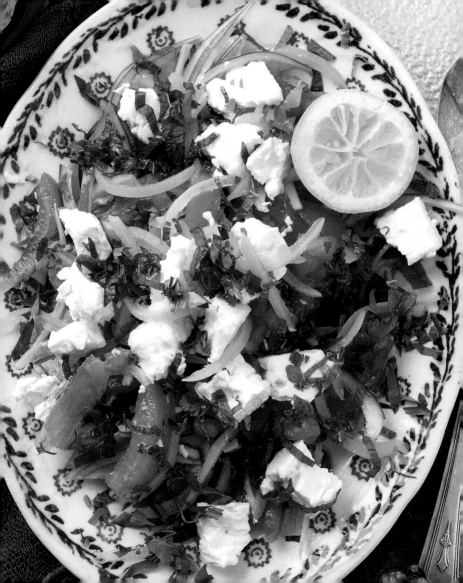

Warm chicken-liver salad

Chicken livers are cheap and good for you, but sometimes they are a little unpopular. Try them in this simple modern salad, and you'll be buying them every week!

TAKES 25 MINUTES ● SERVES 4

140g/5oz fine green beans
200g/7oz chicken livers, trimmed
½ tbsp olive oil
½ tsp chopped rosemary leaves
1 whole chicory or Baby Gem lettuce,
    separated into leaves
100g/4oz watercress
3 tbsp balsamic vinegar

1 Cook the green beans in a pan of boiling water for 3 minutes, drain and keep warm.

2 Meanwhile, toss together the chicken livers, olive oil and rosemary. Heat a large non-stick pan and cook the chicken livers over a high heat for 5–6 minutes until nicely browned and cooked through – they should still be a little pink in the centre.

3 Arrange the beans on serving plates with the chicory or lettuce leaves and the watercress. Add the vinegar to the pan, cook for a couple of seconds then spoon the chicken livers and sauce over the salad.

PER SERVING 83 kcals, protein 10g, carbs 4g, fat 3g, sat fat 1g, fibre 1g, sugar 3g, salt 0.13g

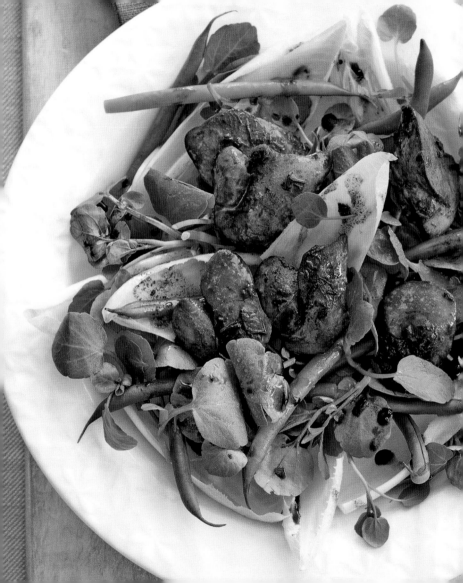

Salmon & egg salad

This is the perfect speedy summer-lunch recipe – so invite the girls over, chill a bottle of Sauvignon and put your feet up!

TAKES 20 MINUTES • SERVES 4

4 eggs

2 × 110g bags spinach, watercress & rocket salad, or baby leaf spinach, washed

12 cherry tomatoes, quartered

½ cucumber, cubed

1 ripe avocado, sliced

4 spring onions, finely sliced

250g/9oz poached or hot-smoked salmon fillets

FOR THE VINAIGRETTE

3 tbsp olive oil

1 tbsp lemon juice

1 tsp Dijon mustard

1 tbsp capers, roughly chopped

1 First, hard-boil the eggs. Put them into a pan of boiling water and simmer for 7 minutes, if you like a slightly runny yolk, or 8 minutes for a set yolk. Allow to cool, then peel and quarter.

2 Gently toss the leaves with the tomatoes, cucumber, avocado and spring onions. Scatter over the egg and flake over the salmon.

3 For the vinaigrette, whisk the ingredients together in a small bowl, adding some freshly ground black pepper, then mix in 1 tablespoon water and spoon over the salad to serve.

PER SERVING 354 kcals, protein 25g, carbs 4g, fat 27g, sat fat 5g, fibre 3g, sugar 3g, salt 2.33g

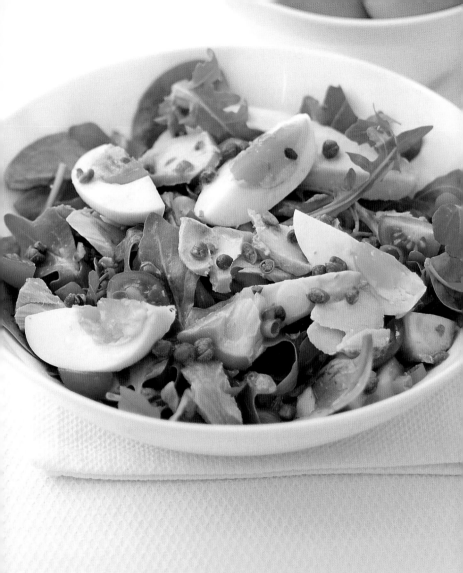

Chicken salad with crisp bacon

A ready-roasted chicken is a clever way to make something a bit special very, very quickly!

TAKES 50 MINUTES ● SERVES 4–6

meat from 1 ready-roasted chicken, shredded
6 rashers smoked streaky bacon
1 small red onion, halved, thinly sliced
2 tbsp olive oil
2 tsp white wine vinegar
100g bag watercress
2–3 heads red chicory, separated into leaves and halved if large
¾ cucumber, halved, seeds scooped out, then sliced on the diagonal

FOR THE DRESSING

200g tub Greek yogurt
4 tbsp mayonnaise
2 tsp wholegrain mustard
1 spring onion, finely chopped
2 tsp chopped tarragon leaves

1 Mix the ingredients for the dressing with a little seasoning in a large bowl. Stir in the chicken and loosen with a little water, if necessary. Set aside.

2 Slowly cook the bacon in a large frying pan until crisp and the fat has run out. Drain on kitchen paper. Meanwhile, mix the onion with the oil, vinegar and some seasoning.

3 Toss the onion with the watercress, chicory and cucumber in a salad bowl, then pile on to a platter. Spoon over the chicken, then break or chop the bacon over the top.

PER SERVING (6) 501 kcals, protein 44g, carbs 4g, fat 35g, sat fat 11g, fibre 1g, sugar 3g, salt 3.12g

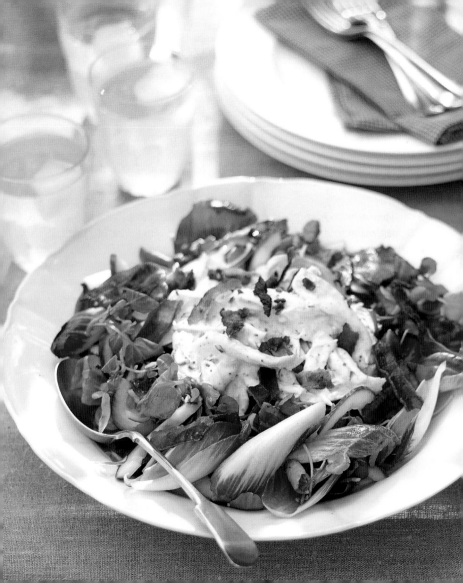

Chargrilled vegetable & mozzarella salad

Don't cheat on the preparation of all the vegetables – the blackening and chargrilling is where all the lovely flavours develop.

TAKES 1 HOUR 20 MINUTES
● **SERVES 6 AS STARTER OR SIDE DISH**

2 red peppers
3 tbsp olive oil, plus extra to drizzle (optional)
1 tbsp red wine vinegar
1 small garlic clove, crushed
1 red chilli, deseeded and finely chopped
1 aubergine, cut into 1cm/½in rounds
1 large courgette, cut into 1cm/½in rounds
2 red onions, sliced about 1.5cm/¾in thick but kept as whole slices
6 plump sundried tomatoes in oil, drained and torn into strips
handful black olives
large handful basil leaves, roughly torn
2 × 125g balls mozzarella, roughly torn

1 First, blacken the peppers all over – do this directly over a flame, over hot coals or under a hot grill. When completely blackened, put them in a bowl, cover and leave to cool.

2 While the peppers are cooling, mix the oil, vinegar, garlic and chilli in a large bowl. On a hot barbecue or griddle pan, chargrill the aubergine, courgette and onions in batches until browned and starting to soften – courgettes and onions are fine still slightly crunchy but you want the aubergine cooked all the way through. As the vegetables are ready, put them straight into the dressing.

3 When the peppers are cool enough to handle, peel, remove the stalk and scrape out the seeds. Cut the flesh into strips and toss them through the veg with any juice from the bowl. Mix in the tomatoes, olives, basil and some seasoning. Drizzle with more oil, if you like, and serve with mozzarella.

PER SERVING 126 kcals, protein 3g, carbs 10g, fat 9g, sat fat 1g, fibre 4g, sugar 7g, salt 0.66g

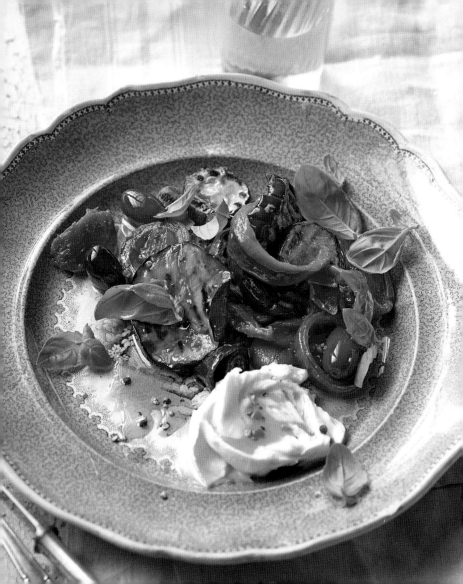

Marinated aubergine & rocket salad

This is delicious all by itself, but for a hit of protein eat it with some crumbled feta or goat's cheese, or a simple roast chicken.

TAKES 40 MINUTES ● **SERVES 4**

2 aubergines, cut into small chunks
3 tbsp olive oil
2 tbsp balsamic vinegar
small handful sultanas
50g bag rocket leaves

1 Heat oven to 200C/180C fan/gas 6. Toss the aubergines with 2 tablespoons of the olive oil and some seasoning in a large roasting tin, and roast for 30 minutes until golden and soft.
2 When cooked, toss with the vinegar, sultanas and remaining oil. Scatter over the rocket just before serving. Can be served warm or at room temperature.

PER SERVING 122 kcals, protein 2g, carbs 9g, fat 9g, sat fat 1g, fibre 3g, sugar 9g, salt 0.02g

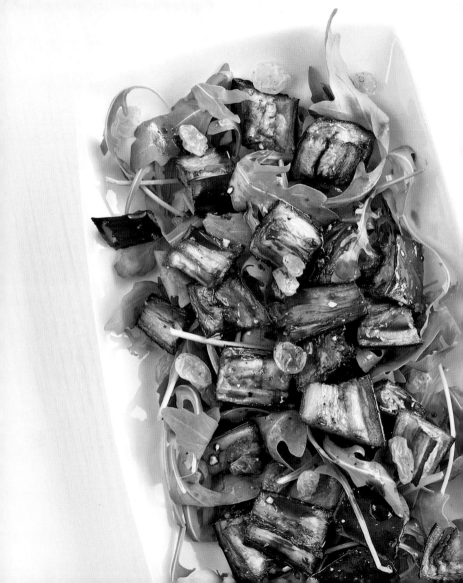

Beetroot & mozzarella salad with maple dressing

This salad is all about showcasing good ingredients. Try to hunt down the special Spanish pickled white anchovies – boquerones – in good delis.

TAKES 1 HOUR 5 MINUTES ● SERVES 6 AS A STARTER, 4 FOR LUNCH

- 4 medium beetroots with roots and leaves
- 2 thyme sprigs
- 4 tsp olive oil
- 2 balls buffalo mozzarella
- 8 boquerones (white anchovies)
- 100g bag watercress

FOR THE DRESSING

- 3 tbsp olive oil
- 1 tbsp maple syrup
- 2 tbsp sherry vinegar
- small knob ginger, grated

1 Heat oven to 180C/160C fan/gas 4. Wash the beetroots, removing any dirt, but leave on the roots and tops. Set aside the smaller leaves. Wrap each beetroot in foil with a quarter each of the thyme, and olive oil and 1 tablespoon water. Put on a baking sheet in the oven and cook for 50 minutes until soft. Remove from the oven and leave to cool.

2 While the beetroots are cooking, whisk together the ingredients for the dressing with some seasoning.

3 Unwrap and peel the beetroots. Cut each into six or eight wedges, then toss with the dressing.

4 Tear the mozzarella into pieces and arrange with the beetroots and white anchovies on plates, then scatter over the watercress and reserved beetroot leaves.

PER SERVING (6) 216 kcals, protein 10g, carbs 7g, fat 17g, sat fat 7g, fibre 1g, sugar 6g, salt 0.9g

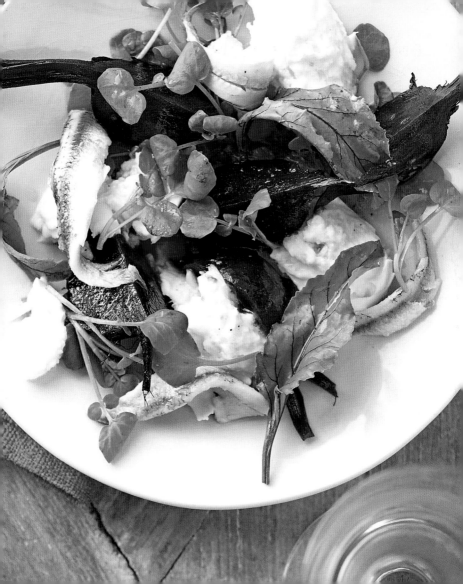

Grilled steak salad with horseradish dressing

A classic Sunday-roast combination, but without the associated carbs! If you like your meat more well done, use sirloin steaks instead, so the meat is still tender.

TAKES 15 MINUTES • SERVES 2

250g/9oz bavette or skirt steak
1 tsp celery seeds, crushed
1 tbsp Worcestershire sauce
a little olive oil, for brushing
6 celery sticks, thinly sliced, leaves reserved
200g/7oz mixed tomatoes, sliced or halved

FOR THE DRESSING

1 tbsp Worcestershire sauce
1 tbsp olive oil
1 tsp creamed horseradish
1 tsp red wine vinegar
1 tsp tomato purée

1 Rub the steak on both sides with the crushed celery seeds, some seasoning and the Worcestershire sauce. Brush with olive oil and leave to marinate while you make the salad.

2 Mix the dressing ingredients together in a small bowl. Layer the celery and tomatoes together. Heat a griddle pan over a high heat, then cook the meat for 2–3 minutes on each side (depending on how thick your steaks are). Remove from the heat and leave to rest, covered with foil, for 5 minutes.

3 Slice the steaks and put on top of the salad, pour the dressing over and scatter over the reserved celery leaves.

PER SERVING 305 kcals, protein 30g, carbs 6g, fat 18g, sat fat 6g, fibre 3g, sugar 6g, salt 0.8g

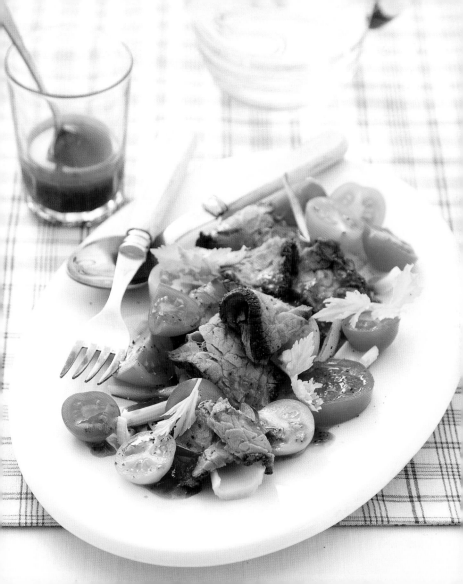

Watermelon, prawn & avocado salad

An unusual but delicious combination – trust us, you'll love it!

**TAKES 15 MINUTES ● SERVES 4 AS A
STARTER OR LIGHT LUNCH**

1 small red onion, finely chopped
1 fat garlic clove, crushed
1 small red chilli, deseeded and finely
    chopped
juice 1 lime
1 tbsp rice or white wine vinegar
1 tsp caster sugar
watermelon wedge, deseeded and
    diced
1 avocado, diced
small bunch coriander leaves, chopped
200g/7oz cooked peeled tiger prawns,
    defrosted if frozen

1 Put the onion in a medium bowl with
the garlic, chilli, lime juice, vinegar, sugar
and some seasoning. Leave to marinate
for 10 minutes.
2 Add the watermelon, avocado,
coriander and prawns, then toss gently
to serve.

PER SERVING 179 kcals, protein 13g, carbs 14g,
fat 8g, sat fat 1g, fibre 2g, sugar 13g, salt 0.91g

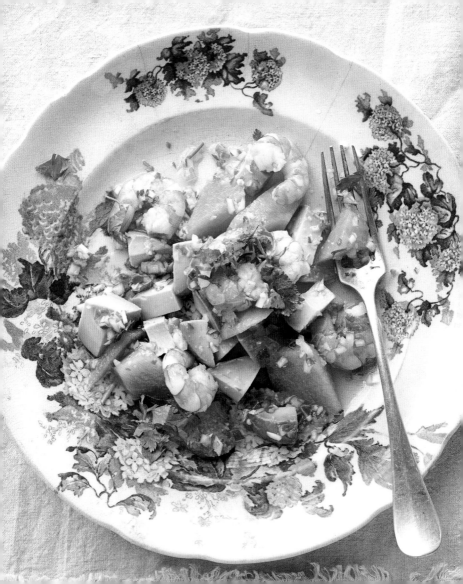

Hot-smoked salmon salad with fennel & lemon mayo

Hot-smoked salmon is a fantastic ingredient, with a lovely aromatic flavour.

TAKES 15 MINUTES • SERVES 2

juice ½ lemon
6 tbsp light mayonnaise
small bunch dill, chopped
1 fennel bulb, halved and thinly sliced
½ cucumber, peeled lengthways into
    ribbons
2 tbsp white wine vinegar
1 tbsp olive oil
40g bag baby watercress
200g pack peppered hot-smoked
    salmon fillets

1 Mix together the lemon juice, mayonnaise, a little of the dill and some seasoning, then spoon into a ramekin.
2 In a large bowl, mix together the remaining dill, the fennel and cucumber, season, then drizzle over the vinegar and oil.
3 Put the watercress on two plates and top with the fennel salad. Flake the salmon on the side and serve with the lemon mayo.

PER SERVING 534 kcals, protein 28g, carbs 11g, fat 42g, sat fat 6g, fibre 6g, sugar 8g, salt 3.8g

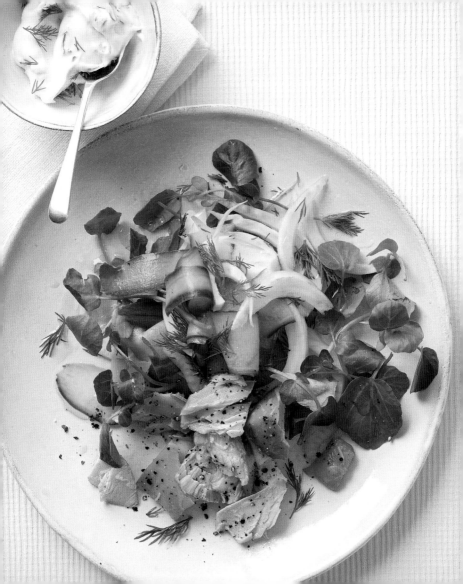

Shredded duck, watercress & orange salad

If you're missing Peking duck and pancakes, this colourful salad will go some way to holding off those naughty cravings!

TAKES 1 HOUR ● SERVES 4

2 duck legs
1 tsp Chinese five-spice powder
5 tbsp rice vinegar
5 tbsp soy sauce
1 large orange, segmented, juice reserved
2 × 100g bags watercress
200g bag radishes, thinly sliced
140g pack chicory, leaves separated
small bunch spring onions, sliced diagonally

1 Heat oven to 200C/180C fan/gas 6. Pat the duck legs dry with kitchen paper and rub in the five-spice and some seasoning. Pour the vinegar, soy sauce and orange juice into a small roasting tin, and put the duck on top. Cover with foil and cook for 30 minutes, then remove the foil and increase oven to 240C/220C fan/gas 9, or put under the grill and cook until the skin is crisp.

2 Remove the duck then strain the juices in the tin through a sieve into a bowl and set aside. Let the duck cool until you can shred the meat from the bones. Skim any fat from the reserved liquid.

3 Meanwhile, gently toss together the orange, watercress, radishes, chicory and spring onions. Pour over the reserved cooking liquid, then add the duck and arrange on a platter to serve.

PER SERVING 248 kcals, protein 27g, carbs 14g, fat 10g, sat fat 3g, fibre 4g, sugar 12g, salt 3.8g

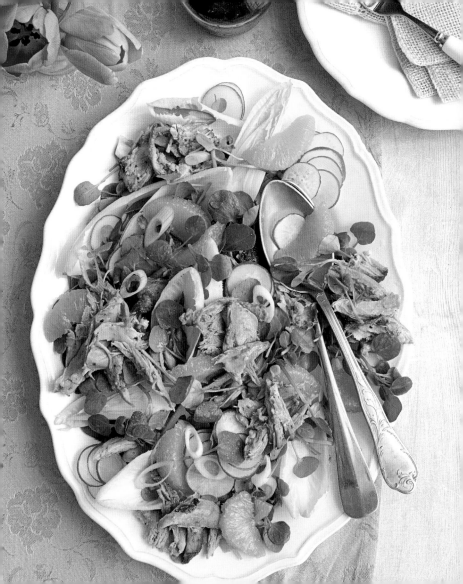

Thai minced-chicken salad

In Thailand, this is known as larb gai. *Chopping the chicken by hand can be a little time consuming, but it does create a much softer and juicier texture than a food processor.*

TAKES 1 HOUR
- **SERVES 4 AS A LIGHT MEAL**

2 lemongrass stalks
4 lime leaves, stalks removed
2 red chillies, deseeded
3 garlic cloves
fingertip-length piece ginger
4 boneless skinless chicken breasts
1 tbsp vegetable oil
1 tbsp sesame oil
1 tsp chilli powder
50ml/2fl oz Thai fish sauce
1 red onion, chopped
3 tbsp lime juice
handful each mint, basil and coriander
    leaves, roughly chopped

TO SERVE
3 Baby Gem lettuces, leaves separated
1 cucumber, seeds removed and cut
    into strips lengthways
200g/7oz beansprouts
lime wedges

1 Roughly chop the lemongrass, lime leaves, red chillies, garlic and ginger, then throw them all into a processor and blitz until everything is very finely chopped together. Mince the chicken breasts into tiny pieces.

2 Heat a wok over a high heat and add the vegetable oil and the sesame oil. Throw in the lemongrass mixture and fry briefly before adding the minced chicken and the chilli powder. Stir-fry the chicken for 4 minutes then splash in the fish sauce. Turn down the heat a little and allow the chicken and fish sauce to bubble together for another 4 minutes, stirring, then add the chopped red onion and cook for another minute.

3 Remove from the heat, pour over the lime juice and toss in the herbs. Serve with the salad, veg and lime wedges on the side.

PER SERVING 261 kcals, protein 39g, carbs 9g, fat 8g, sat fat 1g, fibre 2g, sugar 5g, salt 2.72g

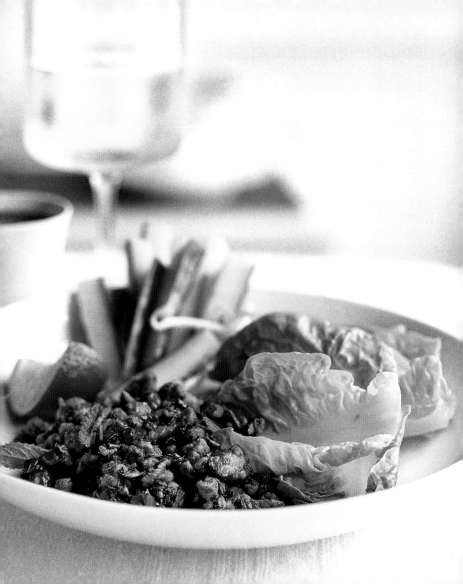

Mediterranean prawn salad

Fish and fennel is a winning combination, which is why this fuss-free salad tastes so great with so few ingredients.

TAKES 15 MINUTES • SERVES 2

juice 1 lemon
4 tbsp extra virgin olive oil
pinch dried chilli flakes
1 red onion, finely sliced
1 fennel bulb, finely sliced
large handful rocket leaves
200g/7oz cooked peeled prawns

1 Mix the lemon juice, olive oil and chilli flakes together. Stir in the onion and fennel with a little seasoning, then set aside for 10 minutes for the vegetables to soften a little.

2 Gently toss with the rocket and prawns, and divide between two plates to serve.

PER SERVING 311 kcals, protein 18g, carbs 8g, fat 24g, sat fat 3g, fibre 5g, sugar 6g, salt 1.6g

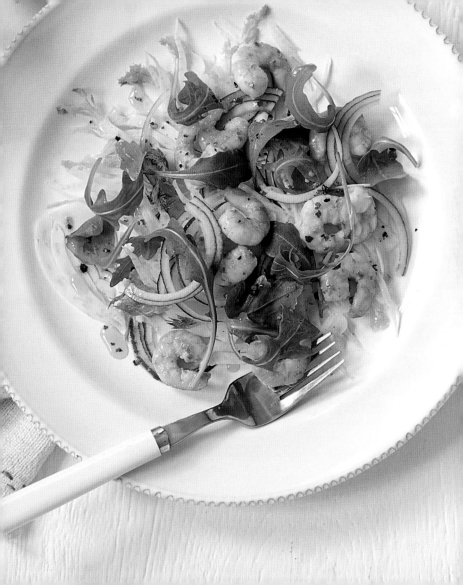

Herby feta & nectarine salad with lemon–poppy seed dressing

This makes a great light lunch, or serve with a crispy roasted chicken for a relaxed summer supper in the garden.

TAKES 25 MINUTES
- **SERVES 4 AS A MAIN, 6 AS A SIDE**

200g/7oz green beans, trimmed

2 ripe nectarines, halved, stoned and chopped into chunks

1 cucumber, halved lengthways, seeds scooped out with a teaspoon, thickly sliced on the diagonal

1 red onion, thinly sliced

small bunch mint, leaves picked

small bunch dill, very roughly chopped

small bunch coriander, very roughly chopped

200g pack good-quality feta

FOR THE DRESSING

juice 1 lemon

1 tbsp white wine vinegar

2 tsp sugar

2 tbsp olive oil

1 tbsp poppy seeds

1 First, make the dressing. Combine the lemon juice, vinegar, sugar and oil with some seasoning. Lightly toast the poppy seeds in a small frying pan.

2 Bring a pan of water to the boil. Add the beans and cook for 2–3 minutes until just tender but still with a bit of crunch. Drain and cool under cold running water, then drain again and pat dry with kitchen paper.

3 Just before serving, tip the beans, nectarine chunks, cucumber, onion and herbs on to a big salad platter or bowl. Finely crumble over the feta. Add the poppy seeds to the dressing and give it a good shake or whisk. Pour over the salad and toss everything together then serve.

PER SERVING (4) 246 kcals, protein 12g, carbs 14g, fat 17g, sat fat 8g, fibre 4g, sugar 13g, salt 1.9g

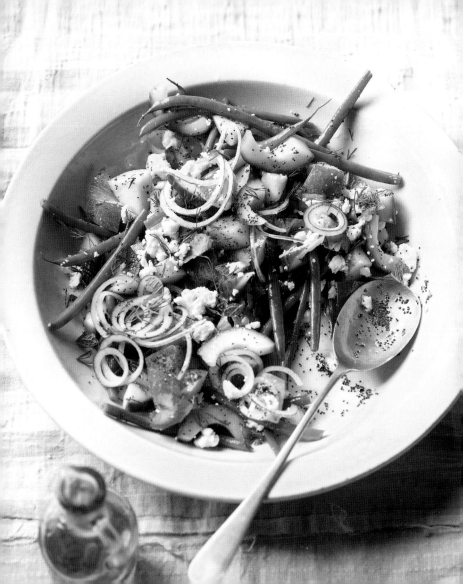

Pear, chicory & blue-cheese salad

Salads shouldn't be restricted to the summer months. This winter wonder combines just a few seasonal ingredients but is packed with flavour.

TAKES 15 MINUTES • SERVES 4

4 small heads chicory (we used a mix of red and pale green)
2 ripe but firm pears, quartered and cored
juice 1 lemon
handful flat-leaf parsley leaves, chopped
50g/2oz walnut halves
2 tbsp walnut oil
100g/4oz blue cheese (Stilton works well) or vegetarian alternative

1 Discard the outer leaves from the chicory and slice in half lengthways. Cut out the base root, then slice into long, thin slivers and rinse. Pat dry and put in a bowl. Cut each pear quarter into three and toss with a little of the lemon juice to prevent discolouring. Add to the bowl with the parsley and walnut halves.
2 Make a dressing by mixing the walnut oil with the remaining lemon juice and some seasoning, then add to the bowl. Toss everything together, then plate up, crumbling over the cheese. Serve immediately.

PER SERVING 284 kcals, protein 9g, carbs 10g, fat 23g, sat fat 7g, fibre 3g, sugar 9g, salt 0.51g

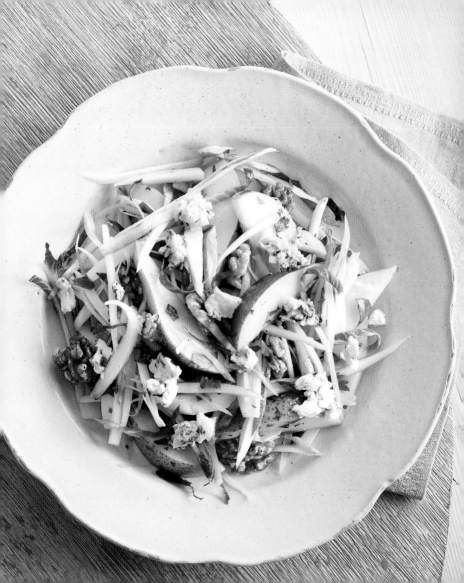

Ginger sweet tofu with pak choi

A trip to the local Chinese has far too many temptations on the menu, so stay at home and cook this veggie dish instead.

TAKES 30 MINUTES, PLUS MARINATING • SERVES 2

250g/9oz fresh firm tofu, drained
2 tbsp groundnut oil
1cm/½in piece ginger, sliced
200g/7oz pak choi, leaves separated
1 tbsp each Shaohsing rice wine and
    rice vinegar
½ tsp dried chilli flakes

FOR THE MARINADE

1 tbsp grated ginger
1 tsp dark soy sauce
2 tbsp light soy sauce
2 tsp brown sugar

1 Gently prick a few holes in the tofu with a toothpick (to help the marinade soak in), then cut into bite-sized cubes.
2 Mix the marinade ingredients together with the tofu. Marinate for 10–15 minutes.
3 Heat a wok over a high heat and add half the oil. When the oil is smoking, add the ginger and stir-fry for a few seconds. Add the pak choi leaves for 1–2 minutes, then a small splash of water to create some steam, and cook for 2 minutes more. When the leaves are wilted and the stems are cooked, season and set aside.
4 Rinse the wok, then reheat it with the remaining oil. When it is smoking, add the tofu (retaining the marinade liquid) and stir-fry for 5–10 minutes. Take care not to break up the tofu pieces and cook until brown on all sides. Add the rice wine, rice vinegar, chilli flakes and remaining marinade liquid. Bring to the boil, reduce the liquid, then spoon it over the pak choi and serve.

PER SERVING 251 kcals, protein 12g, carbs 12g, fat 17g, sat fat 3g, fibre 3g, sugar 10g, salt 3.4g

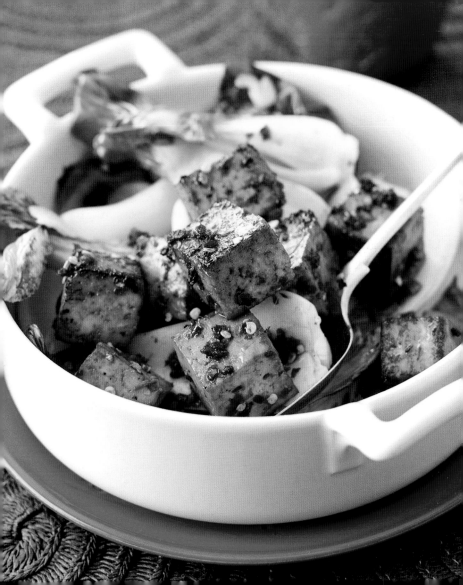

Classic Swedish meatballs

No need to buy in ready-made frozen meatballs – now you have your very own recipe for this classic Scandinavian favourite.

TAKES 35 MINUTES ● **SERVES 4**

500g pack lean minced pork
1 egg, beaten
1 small onion, finely chopped or grated
1 tbsp finely chopped dill leaves, plus
   extra leaves to garnish
1 tbsp each olive oil and butter
2 tbsp plain flour
400ml/14fl oz hot beef stock (from a
   cube is fine)
cranberry jelly and greens, to serve

1 In a bowl, mix the mince with the egg, onion, dill and some seasoning. Form into small meatballs about the size of walnuts – you should get about 20.
2 Heat the olive oil in a large non-stick frying pan and brown the meatballs. You may have to do this in two batches. Remove them from the pan, melt the butter, then sprinkle over the flour and stir well. Cook for 2 minutes, then slowly whisk in the stock. Keep whisking until it is a thick gravy, then return the meatballs to the pan and heat through.
3 Sprinkle the meatballs with dill and serve with cranberry jelly and greens.

PER SERVING 324 kcals, protein 29g, carbs 9g, fat 20g, sat fat 7g, fibre 1g, sugar 1g, salt 0.7g

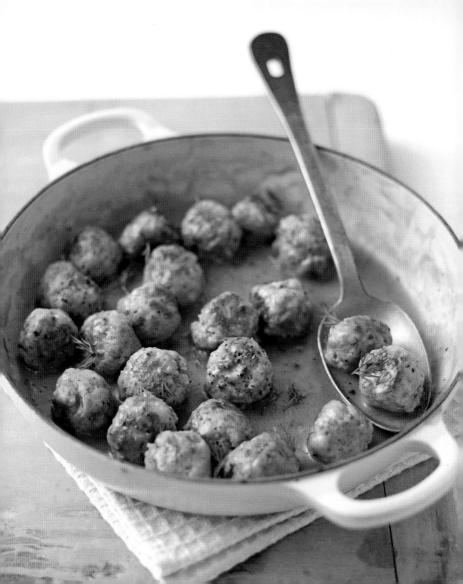

Thai green duck curry

No need to reach for the takeaway menu when you can rustle up something this delicious yourself.

TAKES 2 HOURS ● SERVES 4

1 tbsp sunflower oil
3–4 duck breasts
6 tbsp Thai green curry paste
1 tbsp light soft brown sugar, plus extra to taste
400ml can coconut milk
2 tbsp Thai fish sauce, plus extra to taste
juice 2 limes
6 kaffir lime leaves, 3 left whole and 3 finely shredded
200g/7oz French beans, trimmed
2 handfuls beansprouts
handful coriander leaves
1 red chilli, deseeded and thinly sliced

1 Put a sauté pan over a low heat and add the duck breasts, skin-side down. Slowly fry until the skin is brown and a lot of the fat has rendered off. Flip over to seal, then remove from the pan. Pour away all but 2 tablespoons of the fat.

2 Add the curry paste and sugar, and fry for 1–2 minutes until it becomes fragrant. Tip in the coconut milk, then fill the can with water and add this, too. Add the fish sauce, half the lime juice and the whole lime leaves, then bring to a simmer.

3 Slice the duck breasts, then tip into the curry. Cover the pan, then simmer everything on the lowest heat for 1 hour until the duck is tender. Add the beans, then continue to cook, covered, for 10 minutes until the beans are tender with a slight crunch. Taste and add more lime juice, fish sauce or sugar to season.

4 Stir in the beansprouts for 1 minute more, then serve with coriander, shredded lime leaves and sliced chilli.

PER SERVING 638 kcals, protein 28g, carbs 11g, fat 57g, sat fat 26g, fibre 2g, sugar 9g, salt 2.32g

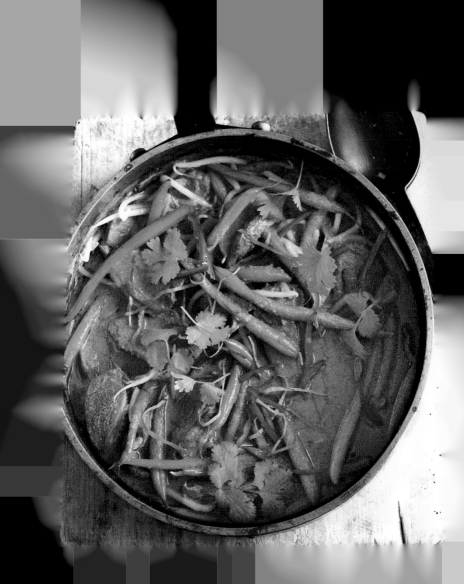

Garlic-butter prawns

Skip the pub and stay in with this absolute favourite – just make sure there are plenty of napkins on the table.

TAKES 15 MINUTES ● SERVES 6–8

300g/10oz large raw prawns, butterflied

2 tbsp extra virgin olive oil

2 garlic cloves, thinly sliced or chopped

1 tsp chilli flakes

zest and juice 1 lemon

2 tbsp flat-leaf parsley leaves, chopped

1 Season the prawns and set aside. Heat the olive oil in a large frying pan. Cook the garlic over a medium–low heat until it just starts to colour. Increase the heat to high, and add the prawns and chilli. Stir quickly and keep turning the prawns in the pan.

2 After 1 minute, pour in the lemon juice. Toss until the prawns are opaque – about 1 minute more. Sprinkle over the lemon zest and parsley to serve.

PER SERVING (6) 73 kcals, protein 9g, carbs none, fat 4g, sat fat 1g, fibre none, sugar none, salt 0.3g

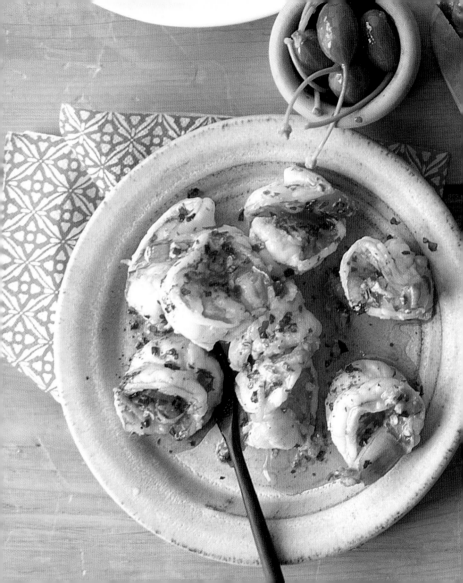

Fish, chips & mushy peas

Who says fish and chips have to be off the menu when you're off carbs? This healthy version is perfect for a Friday-night supper.

TAKES 50 MINUTES • SERVES 4

3 large carrots, cut into thin batons
800g/1lb 12oz celeriac, cut into thin batons
few thyme sprigs, leaves picked
1 lemon, zested then sliced
2 tbsp olive oil
250g/9oz each broccoli florets and spinach leaves
100g/4oz frozen peas
2 tbsp crème fraîche
4 white fish fillets

1 Heat oven to 220C/200C fan/gas 7. Toss the carrots, celeriac, thyme and lemon slices in a large, non-stick shallow roasting tin, with the oil and some seasoning. Cook for 25 minutes, shaking the pan once or twice.

2 Put the broccoli in a pan of boiling water and cook for about 4 minutes or until tender. Stir in the spinach and peas. When all the spinach has wilted and the peas are tender, drain thoroughly. Blitz in a food processor to a smooth purée. Stir through the crème fraîche, a pinch of the lemon zest and some seasoning.

3 Lay the fish on top of the roasted roots and cook for 15 minutes or so more, until the fish is just cooked through. Make sure the green-veg purée is still hot and serve alongside the fish and roots.

PER SERVING 336 kcals, protein 34g, carbs 14.9g, fat 15g, sat fat 4g, fibre 13g, sugar 12g, salt 1.1g

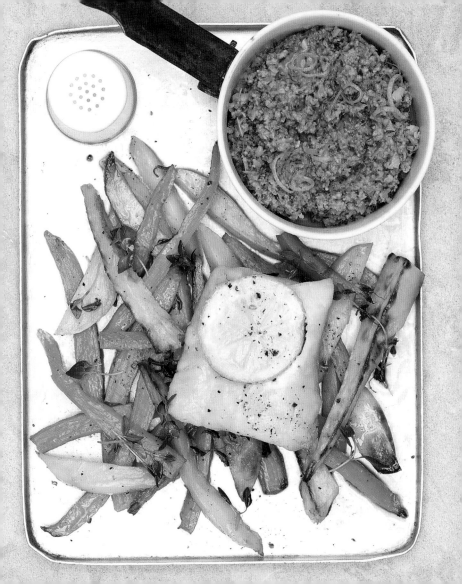

Fajita steaks

If you have time the day before, marinate the meat overnight. This will give the steak maximum flavour and save you time on the day.

TAKES 15 MINUTES, PLUS MARINATING AND RESTING
- **SERVES 4**

4 beef steaks, preferably rib-eye, about 250g/9oz each

FOR THE MARINADE

juice 6 limes

2 tbsp olive oil

4 garlic cloves, crushed

2 tsp dried oregano

4 tsp ground cumin

FOR THE PICO-DE-GALLO SALSA

4 tomatoes, chopped

1 red onion, finely chopped

1 tbsp jalapeño peppers from a jar, drained and finely chopped

2 garlic cloves, crushed

small bunch coriander, roughly chopped

juice 1 lime

1 Mix all the marinade ingredients plus 2 teaspoons freshly ground black pepper in a bowl. Lay the steaks in a shallow non-metallic dish, then pour over the marinade. Turn to coat the steaks all over in the mix, then allow to stand for at least 1 hour, or cover and chill for up to 24 hours.

2 Stir together all the pico-de-gallo salsa ingredients with some seasoning and chill until ready to eat.

3 Heat a griddle pan or barbecue. Wipe any excess marinade from the steaks, then cook for 3 minutes on each side for medium–rare or longer if you prefer it more cooked. Allow the steak to rest for 5 minutes, then cut into thick slices and serve with the pico-de-gallo salsa alongside.

PER SERVING 572 kcals, protein 55g, carbs 9g, fat 35g, sat fat 16g, fibre 1g, sugar 7g, salt 0.41g

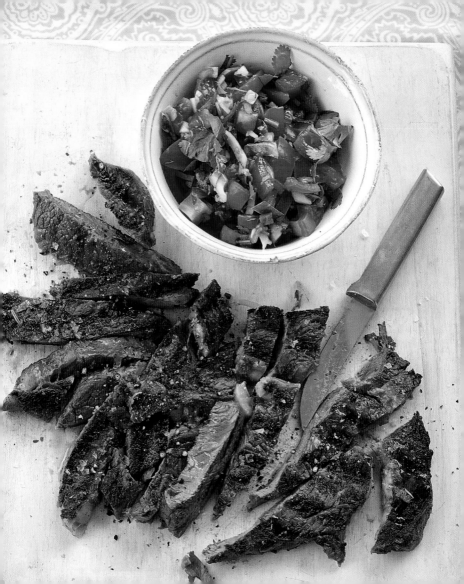

Boiled bacon with cabbage & carrots

Be transported back to your childhood with this comforting dish – perfect for an all-in-one Sunday lunch.

TAKES 2 HOURS 20 MINUTES

● **SERVES 6**

1.3kg/3lb piece smoked bacon

1 onion, peeled and studded with 6 cloves

large bunch herbs, including bay, thyme and parsley stalks, tied together

1 bunch new-season carrots (about 12 in total), scrubbed and trimmed

2 pointed cabbages, trimmed and each cut into 6 wedges

FOR THE MUSTARD SAUCE

150ml/¼ pint double cream

150ml/¼ pint stock from the bacon

3 tbsp English mustard

handful curly parsley leaves, chopped

1 Put the bacon in a stockpot with the onion and herbs, then cover with water. Bring to a simmer, then cook for 45 minutes, topping up with water if needed. Add the carrots, then continue to cook for 15 minutes. Ladle 150ml/ ¼ pint stock into a smaller pan; set aside. Add the cabbage wedges to the stockpot, then continue to cook everything for another 10–15 minutes until the cabbage is tender, but not overcooked.

2 While everything is having its final cooking, make the sauce. Pour the cream into the reserved stock and bring to the boil. Simmer for a few minutes, then whisk in the mustard and parsley. Season to taste.

3 Remove the meat from the stock, reserving the stock, and carve into thick slices. Serve on a platter with the cabbage and carrots, moistened with a little stock. Serve the sauce alongside.

PER SERVING 694 kcals, protein 36g, carbs 9g, fat 57g, sat fat 23g, fibre 3g, sugar 8g, salt 4.51g

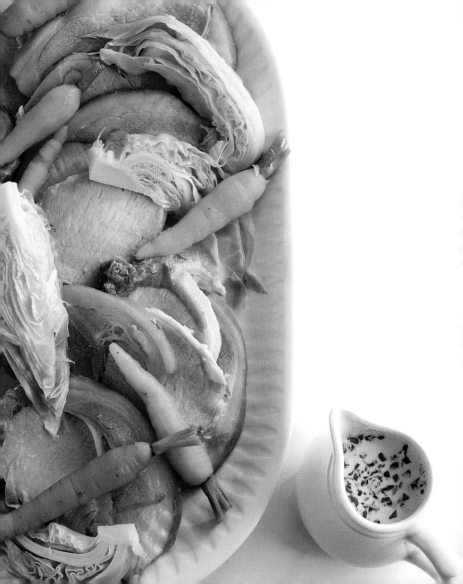

Indian fish curry

Every Friday night should be a curry night; so invite some friends over and chill the beers.

TAKES 35 MINUTES ● **SERVES 4**

2 tbsp vegetable oil, plus extra 2 tsp
2 onions, thinly sliced
8 large vine tomatoes, roughly chopped
4 garlic cloves
thumb-sized piece ginger, roughly chopped
3 tbsp Madras curry paste
165ml can coconut milk
large handful coriander leaves, finely chopped, plus extra sprigs to garnish
500g/1lb 2oz pollack fillets, skinned

1 Heat the extra 2 teaspoons of the oil in a pan. Tip in the onions and a pinch of salt. Cook for about 8 minutes until soft and golden.

2 Meanwhile, blitz the tomatoes, garlic and ginger in a food processor to a smooth purée. Add the curry paste to the onions and fry for 3 minutes more. Stir in the tomato mix and simmer for 10 minutes until thickened. Add the coconut milk and chopped coriander. Simmer again to thicken.

3 Carefully put the fish in the tomato mixture and simmer until just cooked through – spoon some sauce on top and cover the pan if you need to keep the heat in more. Scatter over the coriander sprigs and serve.

PER SERVING 311 kcals, protein 28g, carbs 12g, fat 19g, sat fat 7g, fibre 4g, sugar 9g, salt 0.8g

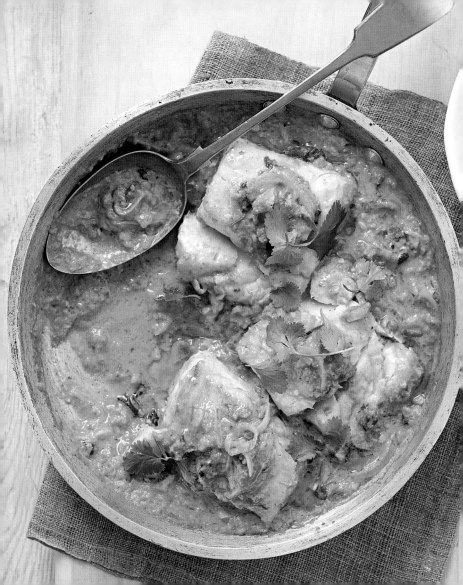

Poached salmon with herby mayonnaise

If you have any salmon left over, mash 200g/7oz with 200g/7oz soft cheese, 3 tbsp snipped chives and the juice squeezed from 1 lemon to make a quick salmon pâté.

TAKES 2 HOURS ● SERVES 10–12

2 salmon fillets, skinned and boned
(about 1.5kg/3lb 5oz each)

olive oil, for greasing

1 lemon, sliced

1 bunch dill, chopped

small fennel bulb, thinly sliced

6 tbsp white wine

1 cucumber, sliced into long thin strips
with a potato peeler

chopped dill leaves

lemon cheeks, to garnish

FOR THE HERBY MAYONNAISE

450g/1lb mayonnaise

1 tbsp lemon juice

6 tbsp herbs, such as chervil, chives,
dill, parsley and tarragon, finely
chopped or snipped

1 Heat oven to 180C/160C fan/gas 4. Take a large sheet of extra-wide foil and brush it with olive oil. Put one salmon fillet on one end of the foil and scatter over the sliced lemon, the dill and half the fennel. Season. Put the second fillet on top. Season and drizzle with the wine.

2 Top with rest of the greased foil and fold up the edges to enclose the salmon in a parcel. Make the parcel quite loose so there is room for steam to develop. Lift the parcel on to a baking sheet and cook for 1 hour, then remove and allow to rest in the foil for 10 minutes.

3 While the salmon cooks, make the herby mayonnaise: mix the mayonnaise, lemon juice, herbs and some seasoning. Keep chilled.

4 Mix the cucumber with some of the dill and the rest of the fennel. When the salmon has rested, transfer the fish to a serving platter. Sprinkle with the remaining dill and garnish with the lemon cheeks. Serve with the mayonnaise.

PER SERVING 559 kcals, protein 26g, carbs 1g, fat 50g, sat fat 6g, fibre none, sugar 1g, salt 0.19g

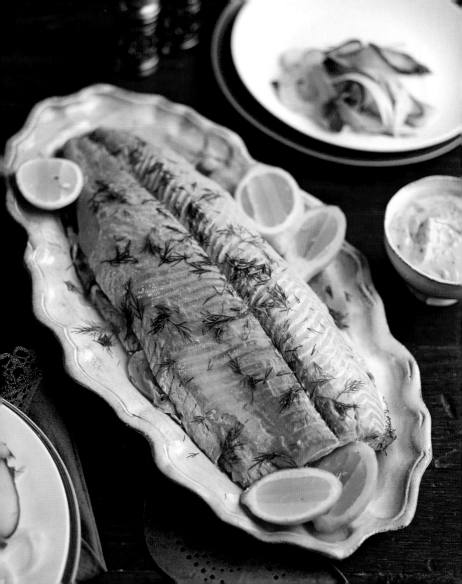

Beef & carrot stew

Sweet, slow-cooked melty carrots and beautifully tender meat – this dish is comfort in a pot.

TAKES 2 HOURS 50 MINUTES, PLUS MARINATING • SERVES 8

4 tbsp vegetable oil
2kg/4lb 8oz stewing beef, cut into large chunks
2 onions, roughly chopped
8 carrots, cut into large chunks
2 tbsp plain flour
2 × 500ml cans Guinness or other stout
2 beef stock cubes
2 pinches sugar
4 bay leaves
2 large thyme sprigs

1 Heat oven to 160C/140C fan/gas 3. Heat the oil in a large lidded casserole dish, then brown the meat really well in batches. Set the browned chunks aside as you go.

2 Add the onions and carrots to the dish, give them a browning, then stir in the flour. Tip the meat and any juices back in, then gradually stir in the stout. Crumble in the stock cubes and sugar. Add the herbs and bring everything to a simmer.

3 Cover and bake in the oven for about 2½ hours until the meat is really tender.

PER SERVING 474 kcals, protein 49g, carbs 14.6g, fat 22g, sat fat 7g, fibre 4g, sugar 11g, salt 0.9g

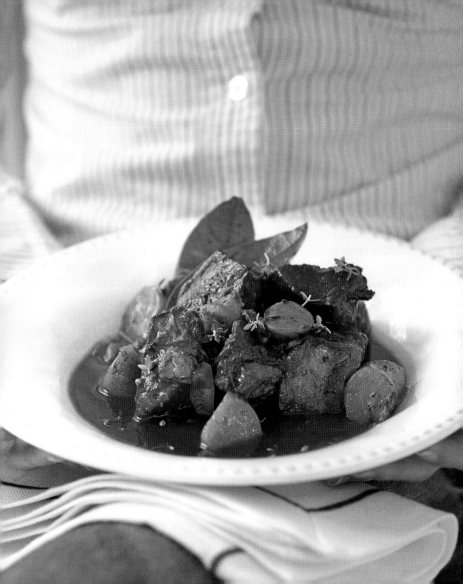

Imam bayildi with lamb & tzatziki

There are hundreds of versions of this Turkish dish, but authentically it is quite oily.
If you prefer less oil, simply reduce the amount used.

TAKES 1¾ HOURS ● SERVES 6

3 aubergines, halved lengthways and
    flesh scored deeply
2 tbsp olive oil, plus extra for brushing
1 Spanish onion, finely chopped
2 garlic cloves, crushed
1 tsp ground cinnamon
8 ripe tomatoes, peeled, halved, seeds
    scooped out and flesh chopped
small bunch flat-leaf parsley, chopped
12 lamb chops or cutlets
pinch paprika
1 lemon, halved

FOR THE TZATZIKI

150g tub Greek yogurt
½ cucumber, seeds scooped out, flesh
    grated
2 tbsp chopped mint leaves

1 Heat oven to 190C/170C fan/gas 5.
Brush the aubergines with a good layer
of olive oil and put on a baking sheet.
Roast for 20 minutes.
2 Fry the onion, garlic and cinnamon in a
little of the oil until soft.
3 Once the aubergines are cool enough
to handle, scoop out the centres. Chop
the flesh and add to the onions with the
chopped tomatoes, then cook for
10 minutes until soft. Add a little more oil
if you need to. Stir in most of the parsley.
4 Lay the scooped-out aubergine halves
in a baking dish and spoon in the tomato
mixture. Drizzle with more of the olive oil
and bake for 30 minutes.
5 Meanwhile, mix the tzatziki ingredients.
6 Season the lamb with salt, pepper and
paprika. Griddle or grill for 3 minutes on
each side, then put in a serving dish and
squeeze over the lemon. Scatter the
aubergines with the remaining parsley.
Serve with the lamb and tzatziki.

PER SERVING 435 kcals, protein 27g, carbs 12g,
fat 32g, sat fat 14g, fibre 5g, sugar 10g, salt 0.27g

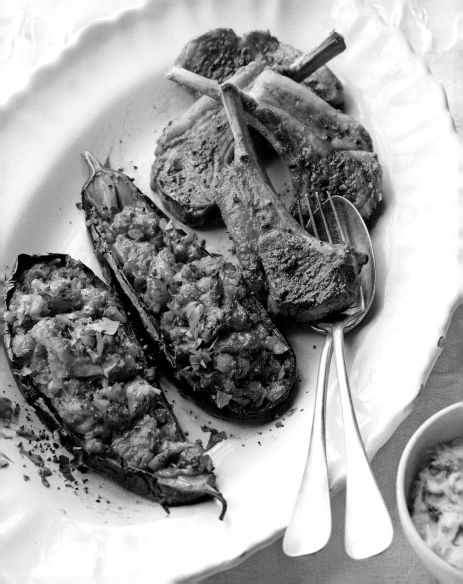

Piri-piri chicken

Everybody loves going out for spicy chicken, but now you can make your own at home – try this on the barbecue and you'll never miss burgers.

TAKES 50 MINUTES, PLUS
MARINATING ● SERVES 4

1 chicken (about 1.5kg/3lb 5oz total),
    spatchcocked
4 red chillies, chopped (deseeded, if
    you don't like it too spicy)
3 garlic cloves, crushed
2 tsp sweet paprika
2 tbsp red wine vinegar
2 tbsp chopped flat-leaf parsley leaves
2 tbsp olive oil
lemon wedges and Tabasco sauce
    (optional), to serve

1 Make a few slashes in the chicken legs.
2 Put the chillies and garlic in a food processor with a good pinch of salt, or use a pestle and mortar. Blend to a paste, then add the paprika, vinegar, parsley and olive oil. Mix well, then smear over the chicken. Leave to marinate for at least 1 hour or overnight if possible.
3 Fire up the barbecue, and when the flames have died down, put the chicken on the centre of the grill, skin-side down, and cook for 15–20 minutes until nicely charred. Flip the chicken over and continue cooking for another 15–20 minutes until cooked through. Check that the juices run clear, as the heat of every barbecue will vary. (To cook in the oven, heat to 200C/180C fan/gas 6 and cook for 35–40 minutes on a roasting tin. To char the skin, put it under a hot grill for a further 5–10 minutes.) Serve with lemon wedges and Tabasco, if you like it hot.

PER SERVING 552 kcals, protein 47g, carbs 1g, fat 40g, sat fat 10g, fibre none, sugar none, salt 0.4g

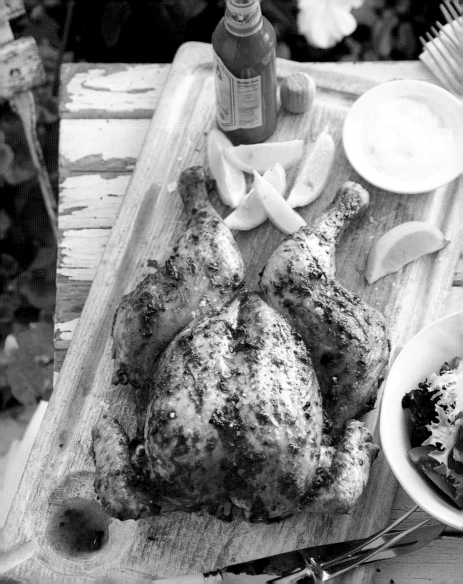

Roast chicken with braised celery hearts

The whole family can eat Sunday lunch together with this juicy roast-chicken recipe.

TAKES 1 HOUR 55 MINUTES,
PLUS RESTING ● SERVES 4

1 tbsp butter
4 whole celery hearts, halved
   lengthways
3 carrots, chopped
4 bay leaves
few thyme sprigs
6 garlic cloves, skin on
600ml/1 pint chicken stock
1 chicken (about 1.5kg/3lb 5oz total)
small bunch parsley, chopped

1 Heat oven to 200C/180C fan/gas 6. Heat the butter in a large, shallow, ovenproof casserole dish and fry the celery and carrots on a medium heat for 4–5 minutes. Add the bay, thyme, garlic and some seasoning, then pour over the stock. Bring to a simmer, then turn off the heat.
2 Sit the chicken in the dish, nestling it into the veg. Season well, transfer to the oven and roast for 1 hour 40 minutes until the skin is golden. Remove to a board to rest for 20 minutes.
3 To serve, reheat the celery and sauce, scatter with parsley and tip into a serving dish. Carve the chicken into portions and serve on a board with the braised celery alongside for everyone to help themselves.

PER SERVING 581 kcals, protein 53g, carbs 8g, fat 38g, sat fat 12g, fibre 4g, sugar 7g, salt 1.2g

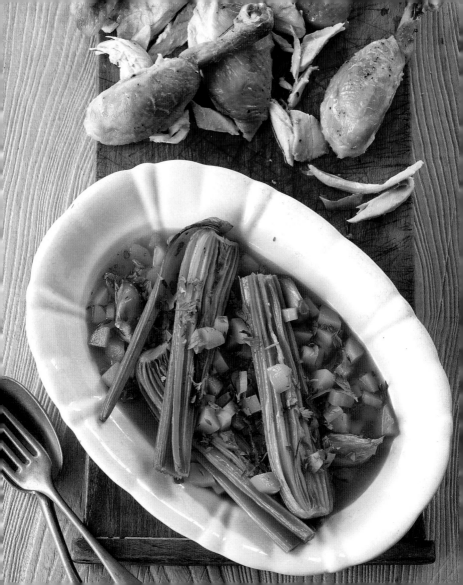

Keema curry with peas

This takeaway favourite uses lots of ingredients you've probably already got in your cupboard or freezer.

TAKES 1½ HOURS ● SERVES 4

1 large onion
2 garlic cloves
4cm/1½in piece ginger, grated
2 green chillies
3 tbsp oil
500g/1lb 2oz minced lamb
2 tbsp garam masala
2 tsp turmeric powder
½ × 400g can chopped tomatoes
   (freeze the rest)
2 tbsp natural yogurt, plus extra
   to serve
140g/5oz frozen peas
small bunch coriander, chopped
shredded lettuce and chutney, to serve

1 Chop the onion, garlic, ginger and chillies together in a food processor. Heat the oil in a large frying pan and fry the mixture until it becomes very fragrant. Add the mince and fry until it begins to brown, stirring to break up any lumps.

2 Add the spices and fry for 1 minute. Add the tomatoes and bring to a simmer, cook for 1 minute, then stir in the yogurt, some salt and a good grind of black pepper. Add a splash of water if you need to, then cook the mixture for 30 minutes. Add the frozen peas and cook for 5 minutes, then stir in the coriander. Serve with shredded lettuce, chutney and some more yogurt.

PER SERVING 394 kcals, protein 29g, carbs 11g, fat 26g, sat fat 9g, fibre 4g, sugar 6g, salt 0.3g

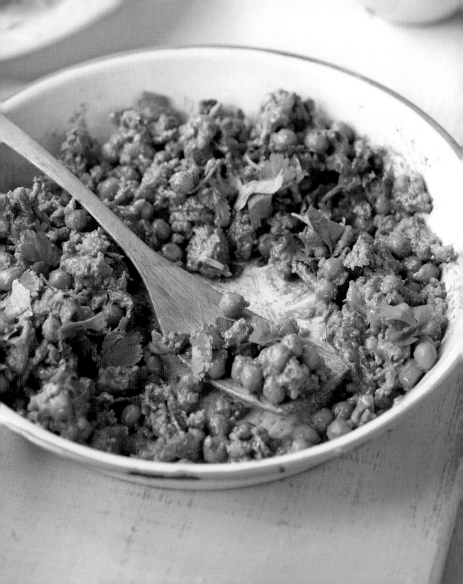

Three-hour pork belly with braised red cabbage

Cooked well, pork belly yields the most beautiful soft meat and crisp, crunchy crackling.

**TAKES 3 HOURS 10 MINUTES, PLUS
MARINATING • SERVES 6**

1 tsp black peppercorns
small bunch thyme, leaves only
3 garlic cloves
3 tbsp olive oil
1.5–2kg/3lb 5oz–4lb 8oz piece boneless
    pork belly, skin scored
2 lemons

FOR THE CABBAGE

2 onions, sliced
2 tbsp olive oil
1 red cabbage, shredded
3 tbsp soft brown sugar
3 tbsp red wine vinegar

1 Pound the peppercorns, thyme and garlic to a paste in a pestle and mortar with some flaked sea salt. Mix with 2 tablespoons of the olive oil and rub over the flesh of the pork. Cover and chill to marinate for a few hours.

2 To cook, heat the oven to 200C/180C fan/gas 6. Rub the pork skin with plenty of salt and 1 tablespoon more of the olive oil. Roast on a wire rack in a roasting tin for 30 minutes.

3 Squeeze the lemons over. Roast for a further 2 hours at 180C/160C fan/gas 4.

4 For the cabbage, soften the onions in the oil in a large pan. Add the cabbage, season, stir and cover. Turn the heat down and stew for 1 hour, or until tender, adding some water if the pan is looking a bit dry. Stir in the sugar and vinegar, and cook for 10 minutes until evaporated.

5 Finally, turn the heat back up on the pork to 220C/200C fan/gas 7 for another 30 minutes. Rest somewhere warm for 20 minutes, then serve with the cabbage.

PER SERVING 625 kcals, protein 43g, carbs 14.9g, fat 44g, sat fat 13g, fibre 5g, sugar 13g, salt 0.8g

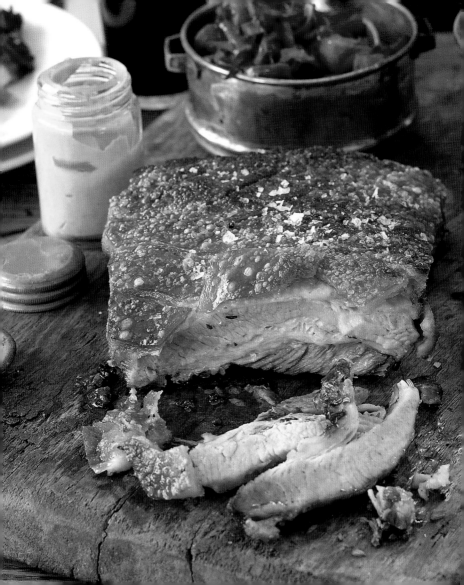

Roast beef with carrots & easy gravy

You might not have tried top rump before, but it's a very economical joint of beef; so it makes a good-value Sunday lunch. It's best eaten pink as this will keep it tender.

TAKES 1¼ HOURS, PLUS RESTING

- **SERVES 4**

1 tsp plain flour
1 tsp mustard powder
950g/2lb 2oz top rump beef
1 onion, cut into 8 wedges
500g/1lb 2oz carrots, halved
   lengthways

FOR THE GRAVY

1 tbsp plain flour
250ml/9fl oz beef stock

1 Heat oven to 240C/220C fan/gas 9. Mix the flour and mustard powder with some seasoning, then rub all over the beef. Put the onion and carrots into a roasting tin and sit the beef on top, then cook for 20 minutes.

2 Reduce oven to 190C/170C fan/gas 5 and continue to cook the beef for 30 minutes if you like it rare, 40 minutes for medium and 1 hour for well done.

3 Remove the beef and carrots from the oven, put on to warm plates or platters and cover with foil to keep warm. Let the beef rest for 30 minutes.

4 For the gravy, put the tin with all the meat juices and onions back on to the hob. Stir in the flour, scraping all the stuck bits off the bottom of the tin. Cook for 30 seconds, then slowly stir in the stock, little by little. Bubble to a nice gravy, season, then serve with the beef, carved into slices, and carrots.

PER SERVING 546 kcals, protein 52g, carbs 15g, fat 32g, sat fat 14g, fibre 4g, sugar 11g, salt 0.65g

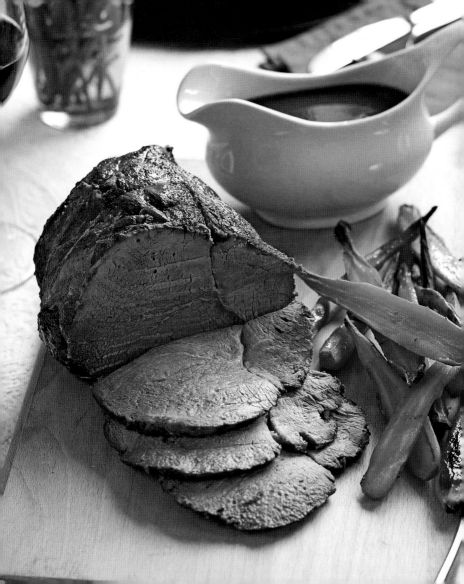

Chicken balti

This curry isn't just low in carbs, it's low in fat and calories too – in fact it's pretty healthy all round!

TAKES 55 MINUTES, PLUS MARINATING • SERVES 4

450g/1lb skinless boneless chicken breasts, cut into bite-sized pieces
1 tbsp lime juice
1 tsp paprika
¼ tsp hot chilli powder
1½ tbsp sunflower or groundnut oil
1 cinnamon stick
3 cardamom pods, split
1 green chilli, left whole
1 onion, coarsely grated
2 garlic cloves, very finely chopped
2.5cm/1in-piece ginger, grated
1 tsp each tumeric powder, ground cumin, cumin seeds, coriander and garam masala
250ml/9fl oz passata
1 red pepper, deseeded, cut into small chunks
1 medium tomato, chopped
85g/3oz baby leaf spinach
handful fresh coriander leaves, chopped, to garnish

1 Put the chicken in a medium bowl. Mix in the lime juice, paprika, chilli powder and a grinding of black pepper, then leave to marinate for at least 1 hour.

2 Heat 1 tablespoon of the oil in a large pan. Tip in the cinnamon, cardamom and whole chilli, and stir-fry briefly just to colour. Stir in the onion, garlic and ginger, and fry for 3–4 minutes until browned. Add the remaining oil, then drop in the chicken to seal for 2–3 minutes. Stir in the turmeric, cumins, coriander and garam masala for 2 minutes. Pour in the passata and 150ml/¼ pint water, then drop in the pepper. Simmer for 15–20 minutes or until the chicken is tender.

3 Stir in the tomato, simmer for 2–3 minutes, then add the spinach and cook until wilted. Season. If you want to thin the sauce, add a splash more water. Scatter with fresh coriander and serve.

PER SERVING 217 kcals, protein 30.2g, carbs 10.2g, fat 6.6g, sat fat 1.3g, fibre 2.5g, sugar 8.2g, salt 0.5g

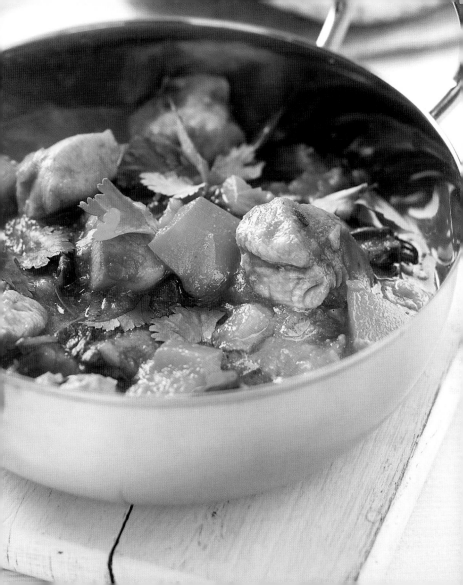

Thai spinach bites

These are great little canapés to munch on before a curry night – packed with flavour, but low in calories.

TAKES 10 MINUTES ● SERVES 4

2 limes
2cm/¾in piece ginger, very finely chopped or grated
1 shallot, very finely chopped
½ red chilli, deseeded and very finely chopped
1 heaped tbsp coriander leaves
2 tbsp peanuts
a little Thai fish sauce
a little caster sugar
8–12 baby leaf spinach

1 Cut a little from the tops and bottoms of the limes so they sit flat on a board. Use a small serrated knife to cut away the peel and pith in strips down the limes. Holding the limes over a bowl, cut away the segments, letting them and any juice drop into the bowl. Squeeze out any juice left in the membranes into the bowl too. Fish out the segments and roughly chop, then drop back into the bowl.

2 Add the ginger, shallot, chilli, coriander and peanuts, and mix well. Season with a splash of fish sauce and sprinkle with sugar.

3 Lay the baby spinach leaves on a platter. Put a spoonful of the mix on each, then hand them round and get everyone to roll them up before eating in one bite.

PER SERVING 36 kcals, protein 2g, carbs 2g, fat 2g, sat fat none, fibre none, sugar 2g, salt 0.15g

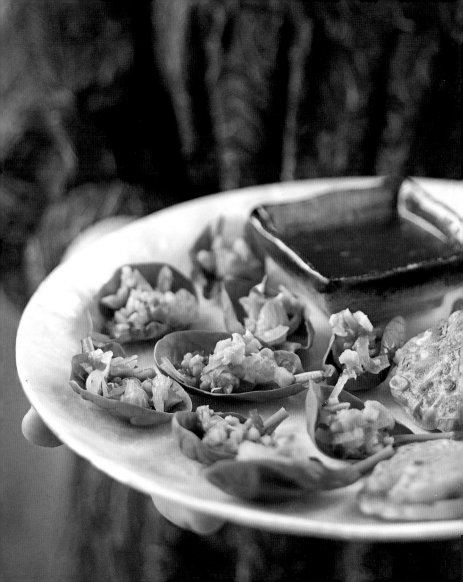

Seared scallops with sweet chilli sauce

Homemade sweet chilli sauce will impress your guests, but if time is short you can always cheat and serve these scallops with bought stuff!

TAKES 1¼ HOURS • MAKES 20
thumb-sized piece ginger
handful coriander stalks or leaves
2 garlic cloves
4 tbsp vegetable oil, plus extra for
   frying
20 scallops
FOR THE SAUCE
1 red pepper, deseeded and chopped
2 red chillies, halved and deseeded
100g/4oz caster sugar
100ml/3½fl oz rice or white wine
   vinegar

1 For the sauce, put the red pepper, chillies, sugar and vinegar in a pan with 100ml/3fl oz water. Bring to the boil, then leave to simmer for 30 minutes until the liquid turns pinkish. Cool, then put in a food processor and blend until smooth. Return to the pan and cook until slightly sticky, about 20 minutes more.

2 Put the ginger, coriander and garlic in a pestle and mortar, then pound to a paste. Add the oil and mix through. Pour this over the scallops and rub in until they are covered with the mixture. Thread each scallop on to a skewer – if you're using wooden ones soak them in water for 20 minutes first. Leave in the fridge, covered, to marinate (up to a day).

3 To cook, heat a non-stick frying pan until really hot. Put a couple of skewers in the pan and cook for 2 minutes, until starting to turn golden. Turn over, drizzle with the extra oil if needed, then cook for another minute. Serve with the sauce.

PER SERVING (scallops only) 51 kcals, protein 6g, carbs none, fat 3g, sat fat none, fibre none, sugar none, salt 0.17g

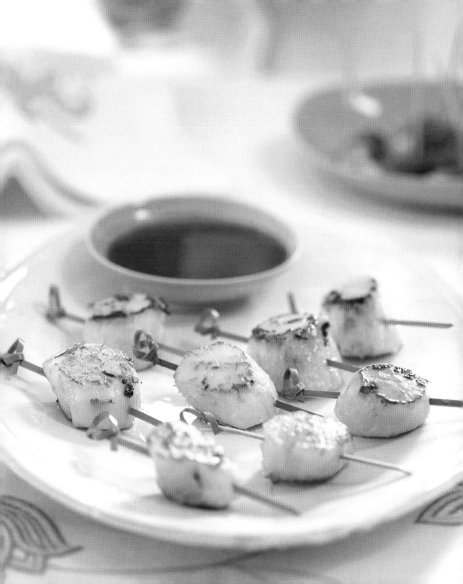

Smoky chicken skewers

These tasty tapas-style skewers work really well as part of a Spanish spread, or serve them as canapés by just frying all the chicken pieces and serving them with toothpicks.

TAKES 30 MINUTES, PLUS SOAKING
- **SERVES 6–8**

6 boneless skinless chicken thighs (about 500g/1lb 2oz total)
2 tbsp olive oil
1 tsp fennel seed, crushed
1 tsp ground cumin
1 tsp sweet smoked paprika (pimentón)
1 garlic clove, crushed
1 tsp red wine vinegar
aïoli or mayonnaise, swirled with a pinch more paprika, to serve (optional)

1 Soak 15 wooden skewers in water for about 20 minutes. Cut the chicken into 3cm/1¼in pieces and put in a bowl. Add 1 tablespoon of the olive oil, the spices, garlic and vinegar, then toss well and season. You can do this up to a day before and chill.

2 Thread 2–3 chicken pieces on each skewer. Pour the remaining oil into a frying pan or rub it on to a griddle pan. Get the pan hot and sear the chicken for 3–4 minutes on each side until cooked through – you may have to do this in batches, keeping the cooked skewers warm in a low oven. Serve with some aïoli or mayonnaise, if you like.

PER SERVING (6) 126 kcals, protein 18g, carbs none, fat 6g, sat fat 1g, fibre none, sugar none, salt 0.2g

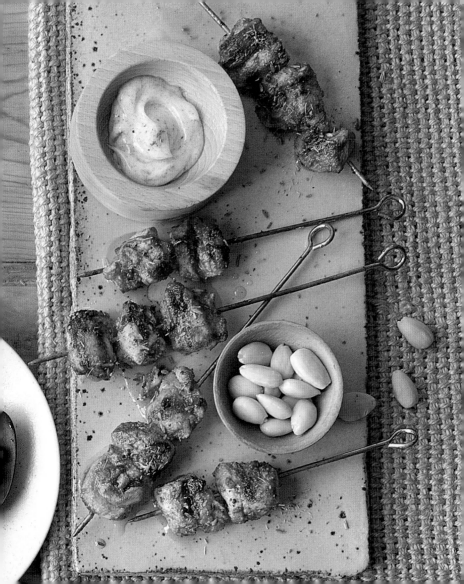

Asparagus mousse with ham & onion salad

Make the mousse up to a day before and leave it to set in the fridge, then all you have to do is top it with the salad and serve.

TAKES 50 MINUTES, PLUS CHILLING

● SERVES 4

1 tbsp butter

250g/9oz asparagus, finely sliced

250ml/9fl oz double cream

250ml/9fl oz milk

1 thick slice onion

handful baby leaf spinach

2½ leaf gelatine, soaked in a little cold water

1 egg white

olive oil, for drizzling

FOR THE SALAD

2 slices ham, diced

½ red onion, finely chopped

2 spring onions, finely sliced

squeeze lemon juice

small bunch watercress, leaves picked

1 Melt the butter in a pan, then add the asparagus and cook until soft but not coloured. Remove from the pan and dry with kitchen paper. Bring the cream, milk and onion slice to the boil in a pan, then simmer until reduced to 350ml/12fl oz – check by pouring into a measuring jug – then add the asparagus.

2 Immediately blend the mixture in a blender with the spinach leaves, then sieve into a clean bowl. Add the soaked gelatine and stir until dissolved. Allow to cool for a few minutes in the fridge, but don't let the mixture set.

3 Beat the egg white to soft peaks, then fold into the asparagus mix and season. Divide the mousse among four glasses and leave them to set in the fridge.

4 To serve, mix the ham, red onion, spring onions and a squeeze of lemon juice. Put some watercress leaves on top of each mousse, spoon over the ham and onion salad and a drizzle of olive oil.

PER SERVING 413 kcals, protein 12g, carbs 7g, fat 37g, sat fat 22g, fibre 2g, sugar 7g, salt 0.58g

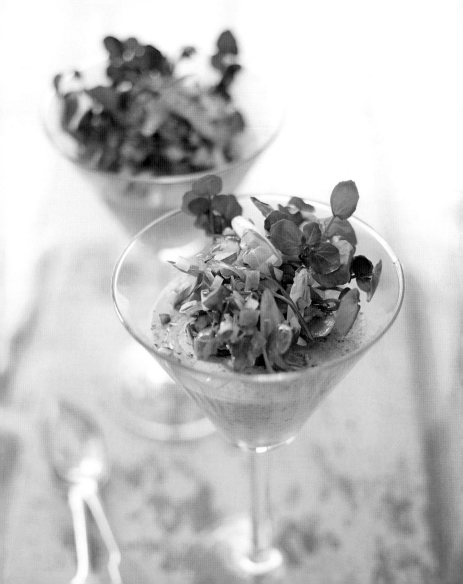

Chicken-liver parfaits

Swap the traditional toast for thin slivers of crispy apple and plenty of chicory leaves as a carb-free accompaniment – perfect for scooping up this delicious classic.

TAKES 40 MINUTES, PLUS CHILLING
- **MAKES 6**

400g/14oz chicken livers
200g/7oz butter
1 garlic clove, crushed
1 shallot, chopped
2 large thyme sprigs
pinch ground mace
good grating nutmeg
2 tbsp double cream

1 Trim the livers of any green bits or sinews. Heat a knob of the butter in a large frying pan and gently fry the livers with the garlic, shallot, 1 of the thyme sprigs and the spices. Fry until the livers are browned but still soft when pressed, and pink (but not raw) in the middle.

2 Tip the livers into a food processor. Whizz to a paste, then whizz in 140g/5oz of the remaining butter and the cream. Push the mixture through a sieve – this is boring, but worth it for a really smooth texture. Season well.

3 Divide the mixture among six small ramekins and smooth the surfaces. Melt the remaining butter in a pan and let the white milk solids settle to the bottom. Pull the leaves from the remaining thyme sprig and scatter over the liver mixture in each ramekin. Pour a little clarified butter over each and chill to set.

4 Serve at room temperature.

PER PARFAIT 336 kcals, protein 12.2g, carbs 0.7g, fat 31.6g, sat fat 19.3g, fibre 0.1g, salt 0.7g

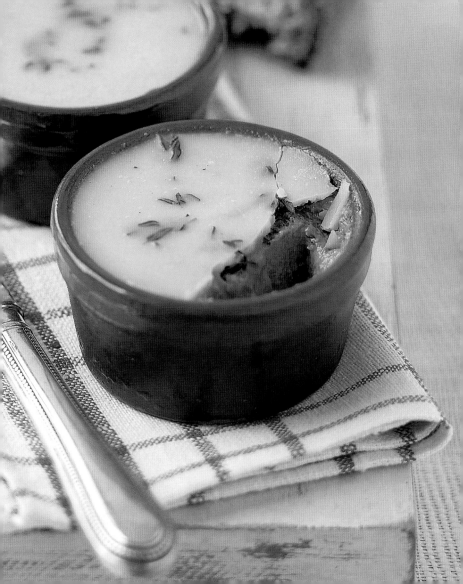

Twice-baked cheese soufflés

These make-ahead soufflés miraculously rise again when re-baked.

TAKES 1 HOUR 15 MINUTES

● **SERVES 6**

1½ tbsp olive oil, plus ½ tsp for
   greasing
1 heaped tbsp polenta
1 tsp butter
25g/1oz plain flour
250ml/9fl oz semi-skimmed milk
50g/2oz Parmesan, grated
1 tsp Dijon mustard
50g/2oz light soft cheese
2 heaped tbsp snipped chives
3 large egg whites, plus 2 yolks
50g bag rocket leaves

FOR THE TOMATO SALSA

350g/12oz cherry tomatoes, finely
   chopped
½ small red onion, finely chopped
1 tsp tomato purée
pinch crushed dried chillies

1 Grease six 150ml ramekins with the oil and coat with the polenta. Transfer to a small roasting tin.

2 Heat the oil and butter in a pan, add the flour and stir for 1 minute. Pour in the milk, bit by bit, stirring. Cook, still stirring, until the mixture boils and thickens. Take off the heat and stir in all but 1 tablespoon of the Parmesan, the mustard, soft cheese and chives. Season and cool slightly.

3 Heat oven to 200C/180C fan/gas 6. Beat the egg yolks into the mixture. Whisk the egg whites to stiff peaks – stir a spoonful into the mixture, then fold in the rest. Spoon into the ramekins. Pour cold water into the roasting tin until halfway up the ramekins. Bake for 15–18 minutes until risen. Cool, cover and chill.

4 Mix all the salsa ingredients together.

5 To serve, heat oven to 200C/180C fan/gas 6. Bring the soufflés to room temperature. Turn each out of its dish and put, right-side up, on a baking sheet lined with parchment. Sprinkle over the reserved Parmesan, bake for 10 minutes and serve with the salsa.

PER SERVING 175 kcals, protein 10g, carbs 10g, fat 11g, sat fat 4g, fibre 1g, sugar 5g, salt 0.5g

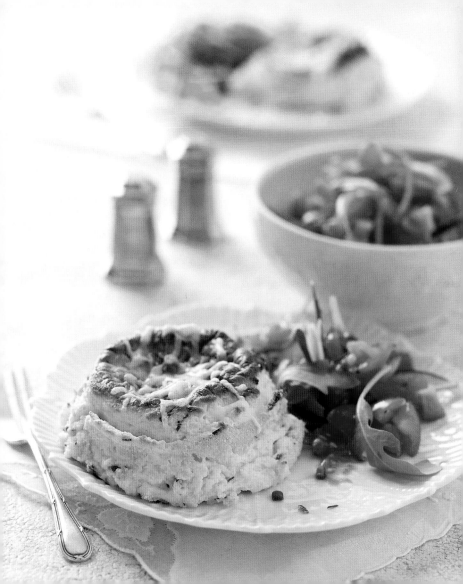

Smoked salmon salad with crab dressing

Quick yet luxurious, this is a gorgeous summer supper to kick off the weekend, especially with a glass of chilled white wine.

TAKES 15 MINUTES • **SERVES 2**

100g tub fresh crabmeat
2 tbsp mayonnaise
good pinch cayenne pepper
½ tbsp lemon juice
1 tbsp olive oil
6 small slices smoked salmon
2 small handfuls curly endive or frisée lettuce
8 cherry tomatoes, halved
1 avocado, peeled, stoned and thickly sliced
1 small shallot, thinly sliced
few rocket leaves, to garnish

1 Mix the crabmeat with the mayonnaise and cayenne pepper. Set aside. Stir the lemon juice and oil together in a large bowl with some seasoning.

2 Arrange the smoked salmon on two large plates. Add the endive, cherry tomatoes, avocado and shallot to the lemon dressing, toss well and pile on to the plates. Top with the crabmeat mixture, scatter over the rocket leaves and serve.

PER SERVING 538 kcals, protein 31g, carbs 4g, fat 44g, sat fat 7g, fibre 4g, sugar 3g, salt 4.5g

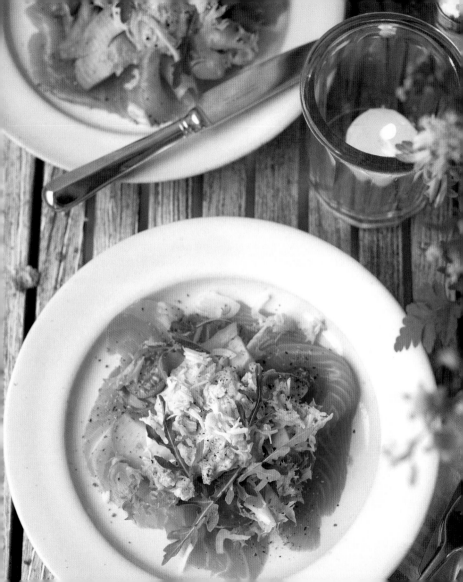

Warm salad of asparagus, bacon, duck eggs & hazelnuts

Get out your best china – good presentation really matters with this tasty but simple salad. Plunging the eggs into iced water stops a black ring forming round the yolk.

TAKES 55 MINUTES ● SERVES 6

6 rashers smoked streaky bacon
3 duck eggs (or 6 large hen's eggs)
500g/1lb 2oz asparagus, about
    30 medium spears
50g/2oz hazelnuts, toasted and
    crushed

FOR THE DRESSING

3 tbsp hazelnut oil
2 tbsp rapeseed oil
1 tbsp cider vinegar
2 tsp smooth French mustard

1 Heat the grill and cook the bacon for 5 minutes until crisp, then snip with scissors into pieces. Cook the eggs in boiling water for 8 minutes (5 minutes for hen's eggs), drain and plunge into iced water, to cool as quickly as possible.
2 Make the dressing: whisk all the ingredients together with a little seasoning. Prepare the asparagus by snapping off the base of each spear – it'll break at the tender point.
3 Just before serving, put the nuts and bacon into a warm oven. Halve the eggs and season. Bring a pan of salted water to the boil; cook the asparagus for about 5 minutes, until just tender. Drain, then divide among plates. Add the egg halves, sprinkle with the nuts and bacon, then drizzle with the dressing.

PER SERVING 261 kcals, protein 12g, carbs 2g, fat 23g, sat fat 4g, fibre 2g, sugar 2g, salt 0.80g

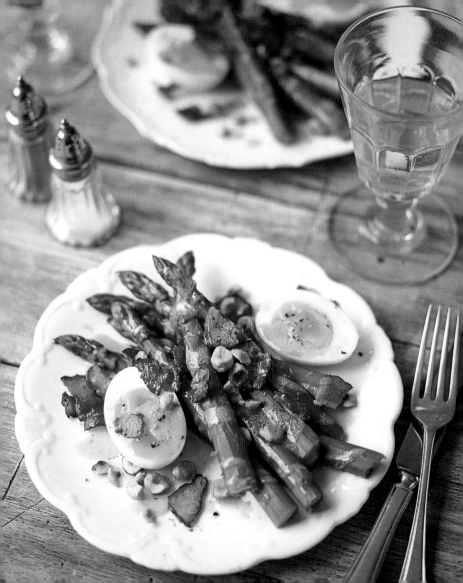

Son-in-law eggs

One story about the name of this dish tells of the mother-in-law who loved her son-in-law so much she cooked him this delight. True or not, it's delicious!

TAKES 40 MINUTES • SERVES 6 WITH OTHER DISHES

10 eggs
75g/3oz palm sugar or light muscovado sugar, plus extra to taste
75ml/2½fl oz Thai fish sauce, plus extra to taste
1 tbsp tamarind paste, plus extra to taste
groundnut or vegetable oil, for frying
4 shallots, thinly sliced
4 garlic cloves, thinly sliced
6 red chillies, deseeded and thinly sliced
large bunch coriander, chopped

1 Put the eggs into a pan of cold water and bring to the boil. Time 8 minutes from boiling. Cool the cooked eggs under cold running water, then peel.

2 Meanwhile, combine the sugar, fish sauce and tamarind in a pan. Heat gently until the sugar has dissolved, skimming the top if you need to. Check the taste, it should be sweet and sour. Adjust with sugar, fish sauce or tamarind if needed.

3 Meanwhile, heat a 5cm/2in depth of oil in a wok or large frying pan. Once shimmering, add the shallots, garlic and chillies. Fry for 1 minute or until golden and crisp. Drain on kitchen paper. This can be done a few hours ahead. Fry the eggs for 3–4 minutes or until the outsides take on tinges of golden brown. Remove from the oil and drain.

4 To serve, quarter the eggs and put them in a serving dish. In a separate bowl, combine the coriander, crisp chilli, garlic and shallots. Pour the sauce and coriander mix over the eggs and serve.

PER SERVING 236 kcals, protein 13g, carbs 14g, fat 15g, sat fat 3g, fibre 0.3g, sugar 13g, salt 2.8g

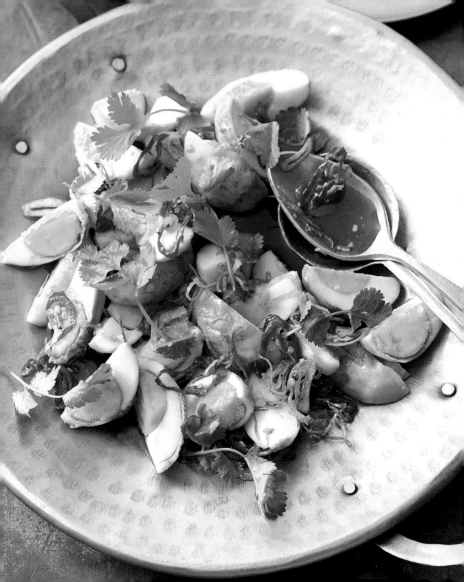

Spanish meatballs with clams, chorizo & squid

Smoky pork meatballs go perfectly with the salty seafood, squid and the spice of the chorizo. All this needs is a glass of something cool, like wine or a dry sherry.

TAKES 55 MINUTES, PLUS COOLING
- **SERVES 4**

25g/1oz butter
3 small shallots, diced
1 heaped tsp sweet smoked paprika
3 garlic cloves, 2 crushed and 1 sliced
2 tbsp dry sherry
300g/10oz minced pork
1 egg yolk
50ml/2fl oz olive oil, for frying
300g/10oz chorizo, cut into bite-sized pieces
300g/10oz cleaned squid, cut into rings
100ml/3½fl oz white wine
300g/10oz chopped and squashed tomatoes (squeeze to a pulp using your fingers)
400g/14oz clams
handful flat-leaf parsley leaves, roughly chopped, to garnish
extra virgin olive oil, for drizzling

1 Melt the butter in a heavy-based casserole, then soften the shallots for 5 minutes. Add the paprika and crushed garlic, and cook for 1 minute until the paprika becomes fragrant. Splash in the sherry, season and cool.

2 Add the pork mince and egg yolk to the pan, then beat well. Shape into 18 small meatballs. Set aside. Wipe the pan, put on a medium–high heat, then add the oil. Fry the meatballs for 5 minutes, just to colour, then lift on to a plate, but keep the oil in the pan. Sizzle the chorizo with the sliced garlic. Add the squid and fry to give a little colour. Now tip in the white wine and bring to the boil, scraping the bottom. Stir in the pulped tomatoes, bring to the boil, then add the meatballs and clams. Cover and cook for 5 minutes until the clam shells open. Discard any that stay shut.

3 Sprinkle with the chopped parsley, drizzle with the oil, then serve.

PER SERVING 747 kcals, protein 50g, carbs 10g, fat 52g, sat fat 17g, fibre 2g, sugar 5g, salt 1.7g

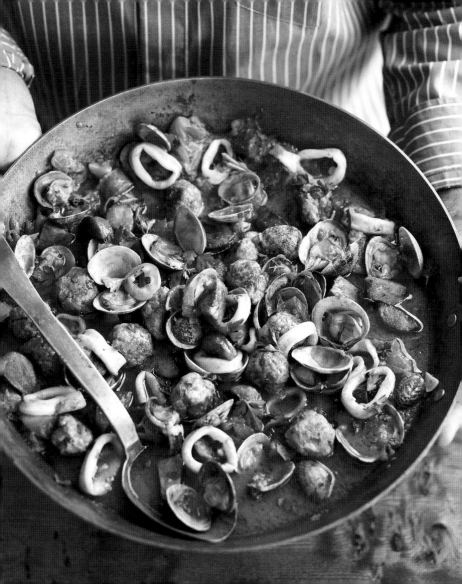

Braised pork with plums

Serve this sweet and sticky delight with lots of stir-fried greens in sesame oil. Pak choi and Chinese leaf would both work well.

TAKES 2 HOURS 25 MINUTES, PLUS MARINATING ● SERVES 8

about 1.6kg/3lb 8oz pork shoulder, cut into large cubes (about 3cm)
5 tbsp rice wine
5 tbsp light soy sauce for flavour, 1 tbsp dark for colour
generous thumb-size piece ginger
5 garlic cloves
1 red chilli, deseeded and finely chopped
2 tbsp vegetable oil
bunch spring onions, finely sliced
2 star anise
1½ tsp Chinese five-spice powder
1 cinnamon stick
2 tbsp sugar (any type)
1 tbsp tomato purée
500ml/18fl oz chicken stock
6 ripe plums, halved and stoned
stir-fried greens in sesame oil, to serve

1 Put the pork into a bowl with the rice wine, soy sauces, half the ginger, the garlic and the chilli. Marinate for 1 hour.
2 Heat oven to 160C/140C fan/gas 3, then heat the oil in a large casserole. Tip in half the spring onions, the remaining ginger and garlic, the star anise, five-spice and cinnamon. Fry gently, then stir in the sugar. Turn up the heat, then lift the pork from the marinade and turn it in the oniony mix for about 3 minutes until the meat is just sealed. Tip in the marinade, tomato purée and stock, stir, cover, then braise in the oven for 2 hours.
3 After the first hour is up, add the plums to the pan. Take the lid off and carry on the cooking, uncovered, until the meat is completely tender. Spoon any excess fat from the surface, then scoop the meat and plums from the pan. Turn up the heat and boil the sauce for 5–10 minutes until reduced. Return everything to the pan, warm through, then scatter with the reserved spring onions to serve.

PER SERVING 530 kcals, protein 40g, carbs 11g, fat 36g, sat fat 13g, fibre 1g, sugar 10g, salt 2.87g

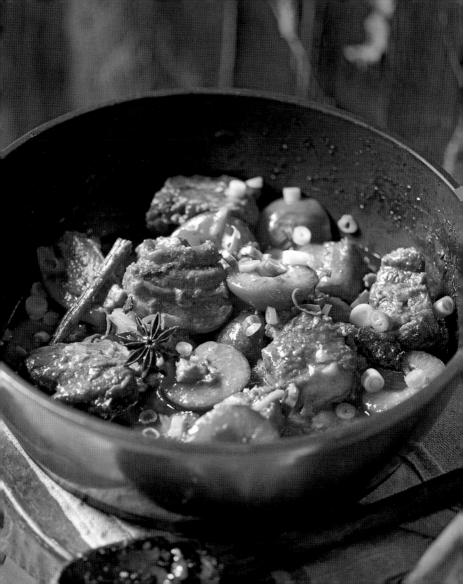

Chicken with sweet wine & garlic

Homemade chicken stock will elevate this dish to something really special, but a bought stock cube will still give a tasty result.

TAKES 1¾ HOURS • **SERVES 4**

2 tbsp seasoned flour
1 free-range chicken (about 1.5kg/3lb 5oz total) jointed into 8 pieces (or 8 thighs, or 4 breasts)
4–5 tbsp olive oil
2 shallots, finely chopped
200ml/7fl oz sweet wine, such as Sauternes
300ml/½ pint chicken stock
sprig each parsley, thyme and bay, tied together with string
1 head garlic, cloves separated but not peeled
50g/2oz butter
200g/7oz chestnut mushrooms
3 rounded tbsp crème fraîche
a little lemon juice, to taste

1 Tip the flour into a large food bag. Add the chicken and shake well to coat. Heat 2 tablespoons of the oil in a pan and brown the chicken in batches. Put the pieces in a large casserole dish.

2 Fry the shallots in 1 tablespoon of the oil until softened, but not browned. Add the wine and reduce a little. Add the stock, herbs and seasoning, and bring to the boil. Pour over the chicken, cover the casserole and simmer for 45 minutes.

3 Meanwhile, put the garlic cloves in a pan with some water. Bring to the boil, cover then simmer for 20–25 minutes. Drain, cool under cold water and peel.

4 Heat half the butter and a splash of oil in a frying pan. Add the mushrooms and fry to soften. Set aside. Wipe the pan and add the remaining butter and a splash more oil. Fry the garlic until browned.

5 Stir the mushrooms and crème fraîche into the chicken. Simmer for 5 minutes, season, and add a little lemon juice if it needs it. Scatter with garlic and serve.

PER SERVING 828 kcals, protein 51g, carbs 9g, fat 62g, sat fat 22g, fibre 1g, sugar 4g, salt 0.81g

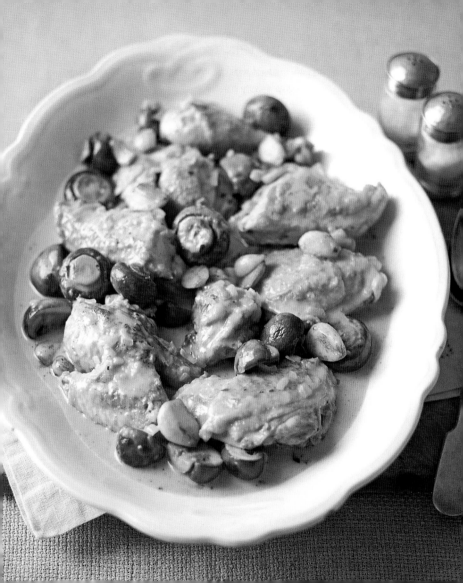

Baked seabass with fennel

Superhealthy and superdelicious – what could be nicer for a romantic meal for two?

TAKES 45 MINUTES ● SERVES 2

2 small sea bass, scaled and gutted
  (ask your fishmonger to do this)
1 fennel bulb, sliced
1 lemon, sliced
handful basil leaves, roughly torn
small handful black olives
1 tbsp olive oil

1 Heat oven to 200C/180C fan/gas 6. Rinse and dry the fish. Season all over, then stuff the cavity with some of the fennel slices, lemon slices and basil. Scatter the olives and any leftover fennel, basil and lemon into a roasting tin. Sit the sea bass on top.
2 Drizzle each fish with the oil and bake for about 30 minutes or until cooked through and starting to brown.

PER SERVING 284 kcals, protein 40g, carbs 3g, fat 13g, sat fat 2g, fibre 2g, sugar 3g, salt 0.53g

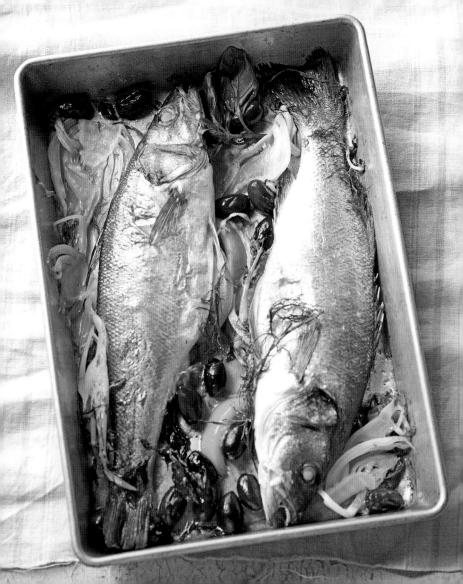

Portuguese braised steak & onions

In Portugal this braise would be served with fried potatoes or rice (or sometimes both!), but it goes just as well with a big bowl of mixed steamed greens.

TAKES 2½ HOURS • SERVES 4

2 tbsp olive oil
4 braising steaks (about 200g/7oz each)
4 tbsp red wine vinegar
3 onions, finely sliced
3 garlic cloves, finely chopped
½ tsp paprika
100ml/3½fl oz red wine
400g can chopped tomatoes
1 tsp tomato purée
2 bay leaves
few coriander leaves, to garnish

1 Heat oven to 140C/120C fan/gas 1. Heat half the oil in a shallow casserole dish. Brown the steaks well on each side, then remove from the pan and set aside. Splash the vinegar into the pan and let it bubble and almost evaporate. Add the rest of the olive oil and the onions and gently fry on a medium heat for 10–15 minutes until softened and starting to colour.

2 Once the onions have softened, stir in the garlic and the paprika. Cook for 1 minute more, tip in the red wine and chopped tomatoes, then stir through the tomato purée and bay leaves. Season, pop the steaks back into the pan, then cover and put in the oven for 2 hours, stirring halfway through and adding a splash of water if needed. Cook until the meat is very tender. To serve, scatter with coriander.

PER SERVING 430 kcals, protein 44g, carbs 11g, fat 23g, sat fat 8g, fibre 2g, sugar 8g, salt 0.46g

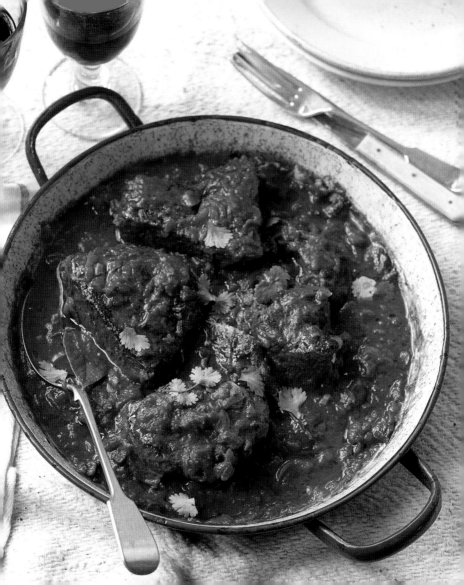

Instant frozen-berry yogurt

Three ingredients, 2 minutes' work – do puddings get any better than this?

TAKES 2 MINUTES ● SERVES 4
250g/9oz frozen mixed berries
250g tub fat-free Greek yogurt
1 tbsp clear honey or agave syrup

1 Put all the ingredients in a food processor (or use a hand blender, if you don't have one). Whizz for 20 seconds until it comes together into a smooth ice cream.
2 Scoop into bowls and serve immediately.

PER SERVING 70 kcals, protein 7g, carbs 10g, fat none, sat fat none, fibre 2g, sugar 10g, salt 0.1g

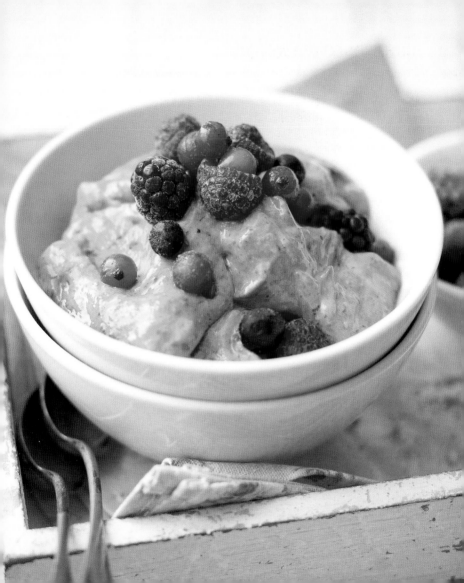

Bitter chocolate truffles

Keep batches of these in the freezer for wowing guests after dinner. For a lighter, sweeter taste, use a dark chocolate with less cocoa solids.

TAKES 20 MINUTES, PLUS CHILLING
- **MAKES 24**

2 × 100g bars dark chocolate (at least 70% cocoa solids), chopped
85ml/3fl oz double cream
1 tsp vanilla extract
cocoa powder and grated white chocolate, for dusting

1 Put the dark chocolate, cream and vanilla in a pan, and heat very gently until melted. Cool, then chill for 90 minutes until firm.

2 Use a mini ice-cream scoop or teaspoon to make 24 truffles, then dust with cocoa or grated white chocolate. Chill until ready to eat. You can make these 4 days ahead or they will freeze for up to 1 month. Thaw in a cool place and, if needed, dust with a little more cocoa or grated white chocolate.

PER TRUFFLE 62 kcals, protein 1g, carbs 5g, fat 4g, sat fat 3g, fibre none, sugar 5g, salt none

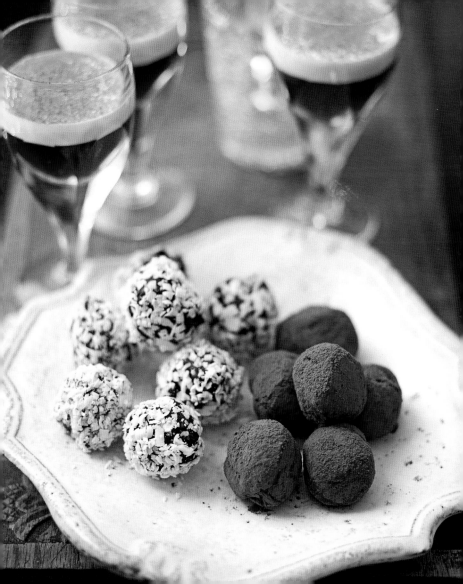

Fromage-frais mousse with strawberry sauce

Making this mousse with cooked meringue not only gives you a light and airy texture but also means you can serve it to vegetarians as there is no need to use gelatine.

TAKES 25 MINUTES, PLUS CHILLING
- **SERVES 6**

1 egg white
50g/2oz icing sugar
grated zest 1 lemon and juice ½
500g tub low-fat fromage frais
300g/10oz strawberries

1 Put the egg white into a heatproof bowl with the icing sugar. Set the bowl over a large pan of simmering water and, using an electric hand whisk, whisk for 5 minutes until the mixture is light, fluffy and holds peaks when the blades are lifted. Remove from the heat, whisk in the lemon zest, then whisk for a further 2 minutes to cool it down.

2 Fold in the fromage frais, then transfer to six glasses or small bowls and chill. Roughly chop half the strawberries and put in a food processor with the lemon juice. Whizz to a purée, then press through a sieve to remove the seeds. Chop the remaining strawberries.

3 Spoon the chopped strawberries over the mousses, then spoon a little purée over each. Chill until ready to serve.

PER SERVING 89 kcals, protein 7g, carbs 14.6g, fat 0.1g, sat fat 0.1g, fibre 1g, sugar 15g, salt 0.1g

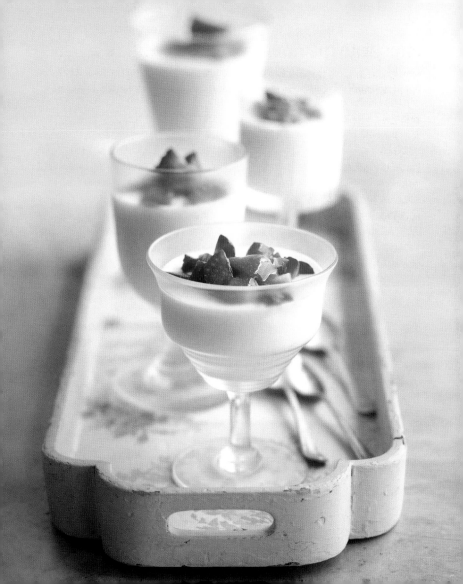

Chocolate mousse

For a lighter pudding, you could use a dark chocolate with less cocoa solids (about 40–50 per cent), although this will make each serving higher in sugar.

SERVES 4 • TAKES 20 MINUTES

85g/3oz dark chocolate (70% cocoa solids)

1 tbsp cocoa powder, plus extra for dusting

½ tsp coffee granules

½ tsp vanilla extract

2 egg whites

1 tbsp golden caster sugar

50g/2oz full-fat Greek yogurt

handful raspberries, to decorate

1 Chop the chocolate very finely and put it into a large bowl that will fit over a pan. Mix the cocoa, coffee and vanilla with 2 tablespoons cold water, and pour it over the chocolate. Put the bowl over a pan of simmering water, give it all a stir, then remove from the heat. Leave the bowl of chocolate over the water, stirring occasionally until melted.

2 The chocolate will be quite thick, so stir in 2 tablespoons boiling water to thin it. Leave to cool slightly.

3 Whisk the egg whites to fairly soft peaks, then whisk in the sugar until thick and glossy. Beat the yogurt into the cooled chocolate. Fold one-third of the egg whites into the chocolate mix using a metal spoon, then very gently fold in the rest of the whites – don't overmix or you will lose the volume of the mousse. Spoon into four small cups or ramekins and chill for 3 hours or overnight.

4 Top with a few raspberries, then dust with a little cocoa powder to serve.

PER SERVING 167 kcals, protein 4g, carbs 15g, fat 10g, sat fat 5g, fibre 2g, sugar 11g, salt 0.12g

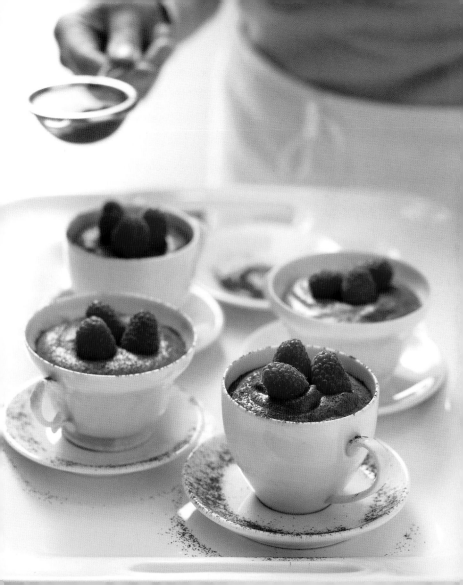

Index

Also available from BBC Books and *Good Food*

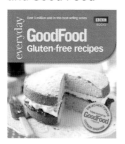
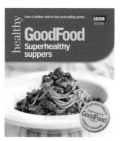

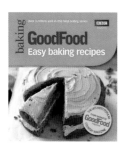
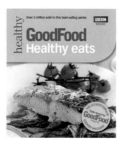

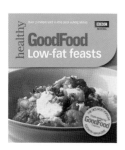
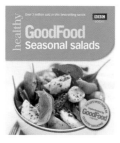

Subscribe
for £10.50! *

Good Food is now available on iPad as a digital-only subscription.

- Subscribe for 6 months and pay just £1.75 per issue, saving you £7.44 on a 6-issue subscription**.

- Each issue is packed with brand-new recipes, including everyday and seasonal meals. Plus get access to the great interactive features of the app – save and email shopping lists, and watch tutorial videos.

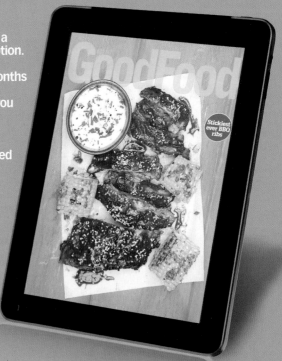

 To get your subscription, and for full terms and conditions, visit *buysubscriptions.com* and click on 'Digital Titles'.